D0301551

Population Health Research

Population Health Research

Linking Theory and Methods

Edited by Kathryn Dean

SAGE Publications
London · Thousand Oaks · New Delhi

First published 1993

SAGE Publications Ltd
6 Bonhill Street
London EC2A 4PU

SAGE Publications Inc
2455 Teller Road
Thousand Oaks, California 91320

SAGE Publications India Pvt Ltd
32, M-Block Market
Greater Kailash-I
New Delhi 110 048

British Library Cataloguing in Publication data
Population Health Research: Linking Theory and Methods
I. Dean, Kathryn
614.4

ISBN 0–8039–8751–X
ISBN 0–8039–8752–8 (pbk)

Library of Congress catalog card number 93–084880

Typeset by Photoprint, Torquay, Devon.
Printed in Great Britain by Biddles Ltd, Guildford, Surrey

Contents

Notes on Contributors

Gerhard Arminger is Professor of Statistics in the Department of Economics, Bergische University, Wuppertal. He is a regular statistical consultant for the Institute of Social Medicine and Epidemiology of the Federal Health Office of the Federal Republic of Germany in Berlin. The main areas of his work include the specification and estimation of models dealing with non-metric dependent variables, latent variables and longitudinal data.

David Cox has been Warden of Nuffield College, Oxford since 1988. From 1966 to 1988 he was Professor of Statistics at the Department of Mathematics, Imperial College, London. He has published books and papers on statistical theory and methods and on applied probability and has been involved in applications of statistics in many fields, mostly but not entirely in the natural sciences, engineering and medicine.

Kathryn Dean PhD is Senior Research Scientist and Director of the World Health Organization Collaborating Centre for Research in Health Promotion at the Institute of Social Medicine, University of Copenhagen. She is also Visiting Professor at the Institute of Public Health, Valencia. Her major research interests revolve around understanding relationships among social, psychosocial and behavioural influences on health, and methodological problems encountered in population research on these subjects.

Scott L. Hershberger earned his PhD in psychometrics from Fordham University. Currently he is a Postdoctoral Fellow in the Department of Human Development and Family Studies, College of Health and Human Development, Pennsylvania State University. His research interests include developmental behaviour genetics and structural equation modelling.

Svend Kreiner is Senior Researcher at the Danish National Institute for Educational Research, Copenhagen. His primary research interests are in item response theory, graphical modelling and exact conditional inference and analysis by Rasch models. He has developed interactive software for analysis of high-dimensional contingency tables by graphical models. He has also developed large-scale Markov chain models, currently used for analysis of trends and forecasting by the Danish Ministry of Education.

David V. McQueen, the founding Director of the multidisciplinary Research Unit in Health and Behavioural Change, Edinburgh, recently assumed the position of Chief of the Behavioural Surveillance Branch at the National Center for Chronic Disease and Health Promotion of the US Centers for Disease Control. His major interests include continuous monitoring of health-related behaviours, new methods and theories for research into behavioural change, and the development of computer assisted telephone interviewing (CATI).

John R. Nesselroade earned his PhD in psychology at the University of Illinois. Currently he is Hugh Scott Hamilton Professor of Psychology and Director of the Institute for Developmental and Health Research Methodology, University of Virginia. His research interests include personality and ability development over the lifespan and developmental research methodology.

Matilda White Riley, DSc, is Senior Social Scientist and former Associate Director for Behavioural and Social Research of the National Institute on Aging, US National Institutes of Health. She is Professor Emerita of Sociology, Rutgers University, and Bowdoin College. She has worked and published extensively in research methodology, communications research, socialization and intergenerational relationships, and the sociology of age. She has held a number of offices including President of the American Sociological Association in 1986.

Nanny Wermuth is Professor of Methods in Psychology, Johannes Gutenberg University, Mainz. She received a PhD from the Department of Statistics, Harvard University in 1972 and a degree in medical statistics from the University of Mainz. Her emphasis in research is on developing methods for the analysis of data from observational studies.

Joe Whittaker, a graduate of the London School of Economics, is Senior Lecturer in the Mathematics Department, Lancaster University. His main research interests lie in graphical modelling. He is a fellow of the Royal Statistical Society, and chairperson of its Multivariate Study Group. He is an elected member to the Board of

Directors of the European Region of the International Association for Statistical Computing, and Associate Editor of *Applied Statistics*.

Fredric D. Wolinsky is Professor of Medicine at the Indiana University School of Medicine. He received his PhD from Southern Illinois University at Carbondale in 1977. He has a long-standing research interest in the use of health services by older adults, and currently focuses on the development of dynamic models of health and illness behaviour using the multiple waves of data contained in the Longitudinal Study on Aging.

Introduction

Kathryn Dean

> Members of the human species do not grow old in laboratories. And universal aging processes must be gleaned, not from studies of any single cohort, but from many cohorts under the most widely varying social and temporal conditions.
>
> Matilda White Riley, in *Perspectives in Behavioral Medicine*

If one needed to identify a single characteristic to describe the dominant thrust at the frontiers of contemporary science, the likely descriptor would be the focus on complexity. Not so long ago, however, dominant views in the scientific community held that research on causation was limited to the verification of observations about specific phenomena according to rigid criteria developed in the empiricist tradition in science. The goal of scientific inquiry was to predict a relationship between a hypothesized cause and its effect. This form of radical empiricism had to be modified after early twentieth century discoveries proving the uncertainty of causal relationships ushered in an era of probabilistic causal thinking focused on predicting the effects of causes within ranges of certainty. Now, however, it is recognized that what appeared to be random variations producing uncertainty in scientific results are actually fine structures arising from complex deviations. The fundamental limits on prediction come not from randomness, but from non-linear structures and from multiple small deviations and interactions among causal forces.

This book is focused on quantitative research involving the collection and analysis of complex information about health issues from population groups. The influences studied in investigations of population health issues are no less complex than those studied in any other area of scientific research. Indeed, we are often faced with far greater complexity. Research on population health issues typically involves the study of statistical associations among widely different types of variables for the purpose of expanding knowledge about human health and behaviour. Results from investigations of this type influence the allocation of public resources and the design of public and professional services. Valid and meaningful findings from population health research are therefore essential for aiding the informed allocation of limited public resources. This means that population health research must operate at the frontiers of scientific knowledge and methodological advances.

The main thesis of this book is that the complexity that is really involved in the causal processes protecting health or leading to its deterioration needs to be reflected in research on population health issues. This raises questions about the role of theory in research and the interface of theory and methods in building bodies of scientific knowledge. Problems that arise from atheoretical research, and the failure to fit theory with methods suited to the research problem, are documented throughout this book.

Many different academic disciplines conduct research on population health questions. Interdisciplinary research on population health holds great promise. At the same time, the wide range of disciplines involved in population health research presents problems as well as advantages. The dominant tendency is still a range of disciplines conducting research, in contrast to interdisciplinary research which builds on the strengths and perspectives of various disciplines working together on the design and execution of studies.

The difficulty inherent in developing and integrating theory and methods in an area of research with many actors, but as yet little truly integrated work, is a barrier to achievement. Nevertheless, the interdisciplinary potential of population health research is one of its major strengths. Many advances in the history of science have come from crossing narrow discipline lines to integrate knowledge or develop new methods. Building on knowledge and theory from different health disciplines has already contributed to the movement away from limited biological to more holistic approaches to health research.

The goal of this book is to pull together knowledge and information not readily available for the purpose of suggesting an alternative to the dominant tendencies in population health research today. We are not providing a handbook on population survey research on health. No attempt is made to present a comprehensive treatment of either the theory or the methods relevant to the knowledge base of population health researchers. Rather we offer an overview of contemporary issues in population health research. This does not mean, however, that the book is only a critique of existing problems in the field. Solutions are discussed and examples of innovative research using newer analytic models are described.

The book is suitable for researchers and students who have a basic knowledge of the methods of survey research and at least introductory statistics. Prerequisite knowledge then includes: a grasp of the options and issues in research design; the theory and techniques of sampling; questionnaire construction; data collection and entry; scaling techniques; a basic understanding of the problems of bias, validity and reliability; and a basic knowledge of the statistical concept of probability.

The material for the book was gathered in a methodological project initiated to draw together an overview of the major scientific issues faced in the field and present newer thinking and options for addressing the research challenges. The Danish Velux Foundation provided a grant to carry out the project. The project was designed to identify methodologists working at the forefront of theory and analytic models for studying multiple influences on human health.

The experts, identified through a process of international enquiries and a search of the literature on research methodology, are highly respected researchers working at the forefront of their fields. With years of research and teaching experience based in traditional methods, they are critical thinkers involved in identifying methodological problems and new options for solving or reducing the weaknesses of traditional approaches.

Papers were solicited from the participants in requested areas of their expertise. The papers were presented and discussed in a working meeting held at the European Office of the World Health Organization in Copenhagen. The papers, revised and expanded as a result of the working discussions and recommendations, form the basis of this book. The chapters take up theoretical and methodological challenges to our ability to expand knowledge about the health of populations.

Contextual Research: Building Theory into Empirical Work

The first chapter is designed to introduce the reader to major problems and issues challenging the field. The discussion focuses on quantitative studies, particularly those commonly referred to as population survey studies. Most of the discussion, however, is relevant for other types of investigations as well. The goal of the introductory chapter is to provide a framework for considering the issues and options presented in the subsequent chapters. An overview of changes in scientific thinking about causation and approaches to obtaining scientific knowledge introduces the issue of facing complexity in research on population health.

The tendency to focus on specific risk factor aetiology is traced to historical developments in population health research and the limits of widely used approaches to study design and data analysis in research on population health problems. The faith placed in experimental design along with the corresponding neglect of theory building and modification inhibit the development of alternative approaches to research on complex problems. These issues are considered in the context of contemporary developments in science. It is concluded that approaches to causal modelling which build on the elaboration of theoretical domains can fruitfully integrate theory and methods to provide new types of knowledge on population health issues.

Perhaps no subject is better suited than human ageing for illustrating the necessary interplay of theory building and multi-method approaches for expanding knowledge in a subject area. In Chapter 2, Riley takes up problems arising from theoretical and methodological deficits in research on health and ageing. Outlining fallacies that grew out of atheoretical research on ageing, she shows us how the forces that affect ageing reach far beyond conventional approaches to research on individual characteristics and behaviours.

Theory serves multiple functions in research on ageing. Not only does it suggest the type of research needed to investigate ageing processes, it guards against fallacious interpretation of empirical results and helps identify substantive areas for further exploration and theory development. Riley illustrates these functions of theory with the paradigm for the analysis of age, a model representing the types of influences that must be recognized in building theory and designing studies in research on ageing.

In Chapter 3, Wolinisky shows how the conceptual logic of the age-period-cohort research paradigm is translated into empirical analysis. To accomplish this, the chapter is divided into two main sections. The first provides a thorough review of standard cohort analytic techniques. The second presents a non-technical review of statistical methods developed to resolve the identification problem fundamental to all cohort analysis. Throughout the chapter, particular attention is given to the need to focus less on technique and more on theory, if age, period and cohort studies are to be successful.

Sound Research: Facing Methodological Pitfalls

Health research on populations often involves the study of causal influences affecting health and behaviour. These influences are generally studied by examining interindividual differences on hypothesized causes in relation to interindividual differences on health variables in samples from populations. This form of variable-centred quantitative research is often conducted without concern for the validity and stability of the variables in the study. This means that variables representing complex concepts may be analysed in relation to each other without concern for serious methodological problems. Chapters 4, 5 and 6 take up design and measurement issues that determine the meaningfulness of analyses of variable-centred data.

In Chapter 4, Nesselroade and Hershberger illustrate the distortions that can arise in research which fails to take into account the variations which occur within individuals on the study variables. They point out, for example, that when the occurrence of a particular health problem is examined in relation to the classification of the sample members on a risk factor, errors may result solely from intraindividual variability in the measurements collected for analysis. Process variables which have particular consequences for the individual's ultimate classification on the dependent variable, they point out, are likely to be overlooked, especially in the absence of substantive theory, owing to the temporal lability often found in the relationship between process and criterion variables.

The authors present both conceptual argument and empirical information which support the value of studying intraindividual variability (short-term, reversible change) as a salient component of individual status on a variety of health-related attributes. Work on the state versus trait distinction in psychology is an example of research on intraindividual variability. In addition to traditional domains of short-term change such as emotion and affect, substantive areas in which evidence of intraindividual variability has surfaced are identified.

Population health research is often conducted on data collected in investigations designed as standard social surveys. In Chapter 5, McQueen takes up design and data collection issues at the very foundation of survey research methods. The methodology developed for survey research is rooted in the ideal of experimental research. Traditional survey methodology builds on concepts and techniques usually taken as given rather than as questionable assumptions or difficult to attain prerequisites. Survey methodology assumes: (1) a well-circumscribed, known (or potentially knowable) population; (2) randomly collected data; (3) the ability to control or assess error arising in the process of data collection; and (4) data representing stable and meaningful constructs.

The meaning and usefulness of the findings of survey studies depend on these assumptions. Technical and practical problems inherent in this methodology are discussed. Newer thinking based on the concept of 'total survey error' addresses some of these issues. A methodological approach for assessing the stability of variables in population data provides options for studying changes in relation to societal developments.

It is quite common in population health research that data reductions are undertaken for the purposes of creating a quantitative measure of a concept. In Chapter 6, Kreiner illustrates that index scales created in these situations can distort findings in the analysis of data in health research if not correctly validated. The validation issues are both theoretical and methodological. They involve both the validity of the scaled construct as a measure of the concept of interest and the possibility that the scale may hide or distort findings about other influences.

Issues of concept scalability and of problems of bias created by scale construction are illustrated by attempts to construct a symptom index to create a measure of morbidity. Since symptom indexes are commonly presented in findings from survey research on populations, this example is highly appropriate for illustrating the methodological pitfalls faced in population health research.

Dynamic Research: Elaborating Causal Processes

Much of today's research is still affected by causal thinking and approaches to knowing developed during the era when positivistic science dominated empirical work. This influence is evident in the pressure for experimental research, or research that approximates as closely as possible experimental design, in preference to approaches that can study causal processes in both epidemiological and social science investigations of population health issues. Central to the main themes of this book – the complexity involved in real causal processes and the need to integrate theory and methods in research that can understand complexity – the chapters on data analysis are concerned with analytic approaches and statistical models that can most readily build theory into empirical work to study interacting and modifying influences in causal relationships.

In Chapter 7, Cox introduces major issues connected with the analysis and interpretation of the results of statistical procedures in empirical research. After a broad review of the role of statistical analysis, the nature of statistical models is discussed. A distinction is made between substantive and empirical statistical models. The superiority of substantive models is illustrated with examples of AIDS and quality of life research. Both of these important contemporary health issues show clearly the complexity of the forces that must be understood in serious health problems.

Theory building around complex research questions requires methods that are capable of specifying and elaborating components of the theory. Not all statistical models are equally flexible and suited for testing theory and using substantive knowledge. Chapters 8, 9 and 10 present statistical models that are useful for elaborating complex relationships among variables, namely graphical models and latent variable models, both well suited for building on substantive knowledge to study complex interactions in the elaboration of a theoretical domain.

Chapter 8 provides a general introduction to graphical models. One of the main arguments against multivariate statistical modelling for studying causal influences is the difficulty of choosing among the multitude of possible models as the analysis proceeds. Model choice determines what is 'found', necessitating theoretically guided decision points. Difficulties of model choice are a major aspect of the rationale for experimental design. However, in experimental design the complexity that constitutes real causal processes is removed, severely limiting the knowledge that can be attained.

As Whittaker outlines in Chapter 8, a strength of the graphical models is that they show how interactions between variables, a cause (or multiple causes) and an effect alter in the presence of mediating influences. The graph, a mathematical statement derived from the properties of conditional independence, presents the pattern of multivariate associations and dependencies in a multidimensional table.

In Chapter 9, Wermuth builds on the material presented in Chapter 8. She illustrates how graphical chain representations of associations among variables can be used to capture essential features of association structures. Following Cox's distinction between substantive and empirical statistical models, substantive research hypotheses in contrast to empirical statistical models are illustrated with examples from health research. A further distinction between moderation in the confounding sense and moderation due to interactions demonstrates the hidden problems in analysing complex health and social data, pointing once again to the importance of theory building and knowledge of the substantive domain.

Chapter 10 provides an overview of concepts and ideas behind the construction and estimation of statistical models with latent variables. Arminger introduces this subject with a discussion of the difference between platonic and operational variables, and describes the rationale for latent variable analysis on the basis of empirical observations fitted into a latent variable model. After illustrations of single- and multiple-indicator models, a conceptual framework for latent variable models is provided. Common latent variable models are described and information on available programs is provided.

Shifting the Research Agenda: Summary and Conclusions

In Chapter 11, the major themes and issues running through the different chapters are highlighted. The implications of new knowledge about the complexity involved in causal processes and changing views about scientific knowledge suggest new directions for population health research.

1
Integrating Theory and Methods in Population Health Research

Kathryn Dean

Introduction

This book focuses on quantitative research involving the collection and analysis of complex information from population groups. Issues facing population health researchers as well as newer thinking and approaches to complex research problems are discussed. A major concern of this first chapter is the role, more accurately the interplay, of theory and methods in population health research. A goal of the chapter is to create a framework for considering the issues and options presented in the remaining chapters of the book.

Two somewhat contradictory tendencies currently characterize population health research. On the one hand, large amounts of data collected in the health sector are analysed only superficially, if at all; while at the opposite extreme, pressure grows for conducting experimental research on population health issues. In the first instance, health information may be simply stored in data banks or summarized in reports presenting frequency distributions. Sometimes the data are analysed in cross-tabulations with or without controlling for the influence of possible confounding factors. When this is the case, a central concern revolves around imputing causation, that is reporting *p*-values or correlations with the explicit or implicit suggestion that they represent meaningful relationships or influences.

Good data, a prerequisite for obtaining scientific results, are only a contributing element to scientific research. In and of themselves, empirical observations, data, do not provide knowledge. The manner in which observations are organized, analysed and interpreted determines what is 'found'. Data collection often receives excessive resources while the analyses needed to extract meaningful information from the data are relatively neglected. Thus valuable knowledge is locked up in large neglected data bases (Glymour et al., 1987). In spite of serious funding constraints for research and the relatively great expense entailed in data collection, this tendency appears to be growing.

An almost polar tendency is the emphasis placed on the experimental model in relation to research approaches which allow elaboration of causal processes and conditions of influence. The excessive faith placed in experimental research stems from the dominant influence of positivistic philosophy and empiricist science during the first half of the century (Suppe, 1977a; 1977b; Wulff et al., 1986). The deterministic view of the world that characterized the era and provided a rationale for the causal thinking behind the experimental model has been challenged by scientific discoveries documenting the dynamic nature of causal processes (Crutchfield et al., 1986).

The central theme running through all the chapters of this book is complexity. The discussion of research issues and methods focuses on the complexity that really exists in health phenomena. It is argued in this chapter that the preoccupation with collecting data that are not adequately analysed and, at the other extreme, the pressure for experimental and quasi-experimental research contribute to the neglect of both theory and the types of methodological issues and analytic options taken up in the chapters that follow.

The relevant background for considering these subjects is an overview of fundamental issues that cut across quantitative health research in the context of general developments in science. Theoretical and methodological issues in population health research cannot be meaningfully considered without reference to general developments in epistemological thinking about scientific inquiry. The starting point must therefore be a review of changing concepts and methods in science generally.

Changing Concepts of Science

The twentieth century has witnessed periods of extreme ferment and change in the accepted meanings of what constitutes scientific inquiry. During the first half of the century the dominant philosophy of science was logical positivism. Population health research, like all other empirical research in this century, has been fundamentally affected by logical positivism (Juul Jensen, 1987; Rothman, 1986; Wulff et al., 1986). Many current theoretical and methodological issues in population health research have their roots in positivistic thinking. Considering relevant aspects of the emergence and rejection of positivism in science is therefore useful background information for examining theory and methods in research on population health.

Logical Positivism

The historical roots of logical positivism are found in the empiricist tradition of the philosophy of science. Philosophical views from that tradition were modified and carried forward by a group which became known as the logical positivists of the Vienna Circle.[1] A range of differing opinions coexisted on specific topics in the development of positivistic science, but any disagreements were secondary to the commonly held view that all knowledge is derived from verifying observations about phenomena (Wulff et al., 1986). The exclusive role given empirical observation had to be modified after rapid advances in new knowledge were achieved through theoretical physics and mathematics (Bohr, 1934; Pais, 1991). The role of theory in the pursuit of knowledge could no longer be denied. Still, the opening made for theory in logical positivism was kept very specific and narrow. The central role of empirical verification was maintained.

Theoretical terms were allowed only as conventions referring to relationships between phenomena. 'Correspondence rules' (Schaffner, 1969) specified the relationship between theoretical and observational terms. The only meaning allowed theoretical terms was specification of observational terms according to the correspondence rules.

The separation of theorizing and empirical verification in logical positivism is found in one form or another throughout the history of empiricist thought. A distinction between knowledge derived from abstract concepts and that derived from the facts of empirical science, originating with Hume (Barrett, 1962), evolved into this cleavage, considered one of the two central dogmas characterizing modern empiricism (Quine, 1962). The second is reductionism, which in the work of the members of the Vienna Circle developed from a radical form of verification of immediate sensory experience to the notion of a range of outcomes supporting the likelihood of the truth of a prediction. These two dogmas, considered by Quine as identical at root, formed the basis of logical positivism. Thus the core of the belief system was built on the view that, in determining truth, only the verification of empirical observations allows one to see if an expected property is present or not, thus confirming or rejecting a prediction about causation. In population health studies, like many other research areas, positivist views influenced empirical research. Hypotheses testing of empirical predictions became the standard approach to research inquiry.

Rejection of Logical Positivism and Subsequent Developments

By mid century many of the major tenets of logical positivism were being challenged. Particularly relevant for the issues taken up in this chapter was the discrediting of the symmetry thesis, which held that a hypothesized explanation occurring prior to an event should be able to predict the event (Suppe, 1977c). In positivistic science, prediction was synonymous with explanation; that is, a causal explanation could only come from a direct test of empirical relations from which a prediction could be made (Hempel and Oppenheim, 1948). Sometimes called the secessionist view of causality, the occurrence of events was explained in terms of expectations based on observations that a specific event will regularly follow another event. The concepts of necessary cause and sufficient cause were used as conventional terminology to discuss causal relationships: if Y is always preceded by X, then X is a necessary cause of Y; if Y always succeeds X, then X is a sufficient cause of Y.[2]

The symmetry thesis became a major subject of debate among critics and defenders of the major tenets of positivism (Scriven, 1962; Wilson, 1967). Various examples illustrated that predictions did not provide explanations, and that theories could provide explanations without providing predictions, notably evolutionary theory (Toulmin, 1961). Furthermore, it was shown that the symmetry thesis would accept explanations which proved to be spurious, dependent on the initial conditions selected in an experiment (Bromberger, 1966).

Parallel with the challenges to specific tenets of logical positivism, alternative epistemologies were developed which totally rejected the doctrine as a viable approach to knowing. One of the more influential alternative views in relation to the issues taken up in this chapter is the falsification doctrine of Karl Popper (1965). Popper rejected the dominant role given to observation in positivistic science. He maintained that the idea of starting the scientific process with observations unguided by theory is absurd. Grounded in the arguments of David Hume against inductive reasoning, Popper holds that scientific theories can only be empirically falsified. The accumulation of observational evidence can never prove a theory, but failed attempts to falsify a theory provide support for its truth. In this approach, science involves the generation and refutation of hypotheses about the occurrence of phenomena. The formulation of hypotheses precedes observations of relationships between events in a 'method of trial and error – of conjecture and refutation' (Popper, 1965: 51).

Popper's views, put forth as an option to the weaknesses of inductive verification, in turn became the subject of convincing criticisms (Putnam, 1971; Faust, 1984; Pearce, 1990). Since Popper's philosophical approach to the accumulation of knowledge was adopted in epidemiology (Rothman, 1986; Weed, 1986; Maclure, 1985), these criticisms figure in current debates about the epistemological basis of epidemiology, and for our purposes are best taken up in that context.

Another challenge to logical positivism focused on science as a social enterprise, totally rejecting the distinction between theory and observation built into the doctrine that science is confirmation and justification of empirical observations. As a well-known proponent of this tradition, Kuhn (1962) described a process by which a 'scientific paradigm' governs the thinking and approach to knowledge in a given discipline. In this thinking science can only be understood in developmental terms: which experiments are chosen, which theories are accepted or rejected, and how theories are used in the sociopolitical context of the time. Theories which do not meet the criteria for acceptance are generally modified within the bounds of the common methodologies and other interests of scientists in a field.

According to Kuhn, periods of 'normal' science characterized by a community of scientists agreeing about research questions, theories, methods and approaches dominate until unsolved problems introduce periods of doubt, ultimately leading to a scientific revolution. In this view, alternative theories and methods, around which new communities form, produce new periods of normal science.

These views, popular in some circles, were criticized among philosophers of science because of the extreme subjectiveness of the doctrines which precluded any rational basis for the comparison of theories (Shapere, 1964). A major criticism of Kuhn's concept of normal science is that it reduces knowledge to the joint prejudices of scientists who agree on the same theory and methods (Suppe, 1977a).

Causal Thinking in Population Health Research: Remnants of Positivism

Population health research draws on the theories and methods of many disciplines. This reflects new thinking and knowledge about the range of influences shaping health. Over the past few decades the biomedical mechanical model of disease, which dominated the scientific paradigm guiding research on human health during the first half of this century, has been increasingly questioned (Wulff et al., 1986). Important research findings in the fields of epidemiology, occupational health, social medicine and sociology are building new bodies of knowledge about the role of environmental and social influences in health maintenance and promotion. Generalizations about concepts of causality in the different disciplines would oversimplify the diverse approaches to obtaining knowledge about causal relationships. It is possible, however, to consider major developments in the most commonly used methodological approaches to quantitative research on population health issues.

Risk Factor Research on Population Health Issues

The currently dominant paradigm in research on population health builds on the epidemiological concept of risk of disease occurrence. Risk factor research is based on one type of probabilistic thinking and methods developed after the scientific advances which led to the rejection of classical determinism in science. Beliefs about simple sequences of causes and effects were no longer tenable after discoveries proving fundamental uncertainty in the occurrence of phenomena (Bohr, 1934; Heisenberg, 1958).

With roots in infectious disease epidemiology and the germ theory of disease, the risk factor research tradition focuses on specific risks associated with specific diseases (Duncan, 1988). Germ theory had emerged and become the dominant theory of disease after important nineteenth century discoveries, especially those of Pasteur and Koch, identifying micro-organisms associated with the serious diseases of that time (Rosen, 1958). Evidence of serious weaknesses in germ theory were soon evident. Koch developed four criteria for the establishment of a causal relationship between a micro-organism and a disease: (1) evidence of the presence of a particular organism in each case of the disease; (2) the absence of the organism in question in any other disease; (3) the isolation of the micro-organism in cultures; and (4) the ability to cause the disease to occur again with the cultured organism.

Koch's fourth postulate was a stumbling block from the start. He was never able to cause the disease to appear with the cultured organism. It turned out that the difficulty was not limited to the fact that the organism he was working with, the cholera bacillus, can live only in man. The problem arose from the fundamental weakness of germ theory; the focus on single causes and specific aetiology. The simple linking of infection with disease in germ theory was shown to be an untenable causal theory (Duncan, 1988; Dubos, 1965).

Theories of susceptibility have long replaced the simpler notions of germ theory. Today it is recognized that the relative capacity of an infectious agent to overcome available host defences is determined by complex processes involving variations in both the disease agent and the host. Normal host defences function to protect the individual from the multitude of disease producing organisms to which there is constant exposure. Persons who are 'immuno-compromised', however, may be infected by relatively benign organisms. This means that 'minor alterations of host defenses may create major differences in apparent virulence of some pathogens' (Sparling, 1983). This is referred to as host susceptibility.

The field of epidemiology was built on recognition of multilevel causal influences on health. Disease patterns in populations were studied in relation to host, agent and environmental influences (Fox et al., 1970; Lilienfield and Lilienfield, 1980; Duncan, 1988). Host factors thus constituted one of the cornerstones of classical epidemiology. In spite of the documented complexity of disease processes, the dominant focus is usually on disease agents (now extended to include a wide range of non-infectious factors), with host resistance considered only indirectly if at all.

Suspected aetiological factors are studied in a framework of relative occurrence of specific outcomes in the presence or absence of the hypothesized causal factor. The occurrence of disease (disability/death) is assessed on the basis of a two-stage sequence of reasoning. A statistical association is established between agent/behaviour/characteristic and the outcome variable. Thereafter, biological inferences are derived from the pattern of statistical associations. Two questions guide the research. Have persons with the disease under study more frequently been exposed to the agent (behaviour/characteristic) than those without the disease? Do persons with or exposed to the factor under study develop the disease more frequently than those without exposure (Lilienfield and Lilienfield, 1980)?

A major goal of contemporary epidemiology is to achieve standards of experimentation in order to infer effect estimates for causal factors. Experimental design and its approximations are based on the principle of controlling extraneous factors in order to observe the effects of the study factor. The goal is to create circumstances in which the variation of extraneous factors is kept small in relation to the variation of the factor under study in order to generalize information from controlled empirical observations to abstract knowledge. This is an empiricist approach to causal inquiry which, as reflected in the following quotation, aims to establish general and universal conclusions by observing causal relationships:

> In science the generalization from the actual study experience is not made to a population of which the study experience is a sample in a technical sense of probability sampling. Such statistical sample-to-

> population inference (generalization) is characteristic of particularistic research only – where parameters of a *particularistic population* are the targets of inference. In science the generalization is from the actual study experience to the abstract, with no referent in place or time. (Miettinen, 1985: 47)

Verification Issues in Contemporary Epidemiology

Rothman (1986), attempting to avoid the inadequacies of inductive verification in epidemiological research, developed a model for the investigation of disease occurrence in populations based on Popper's approach to the accumulation of knowledge by the falsification of hypotheses. Deductive logic is used to develop hypotheses which are tested by comparing observations with predictions. The falsification doctrine thus attempts to sidestep problems in probabilistic empirical induction by negating rather than verifying hypotheses.

Rothman modifies the traditional concepts of necessary and sufficient conditions in empiricist science, and uses the terms 'sufficient cause' and 'component causes'. Sufficient cause is defined as a set of minimal conditions and events that inevitably produce disease. The concept of sufficient cause, in turn, builds on the presence of component causes. Constellations of component causes produce the disease. Each constellation constitutes a sufficient cause. It is unclear how the constellations of component causes are to be studied to arrive at a sufficient cause. The methodology developed to study causal effects by falsifying hypotheses attempts to deal with the problem of confounding among causal influences in the study design by random allocation of sample members. This approach to causal research focuses on the impact of one factor, by shutting out moderating and multiple influences. If random allocation or comparable control groups are not attainable, then stratification or multivariate statistical analysis is used to control for possible confounding factors.[3]

The usefulness of Rothman's falsification methods depends on the ability to elaborate component causes, and on the adequacy of Popper's falsification approach. Since the mid 1980s these issues have been subjects of debate. Among the proponents of the doctrine of falsification, Weed (1986) emphasized that the fundamental scientific problem for epidemiology is how to propose and test causal hypotheses. Contrasting inductive and deductive inference, he argued that epidemiology has neglected deductive logic. Similarly, Maclure (1985), contrasting in detail verification and refutation, criticized the faith placed in estimates based on confidence intervals as the 'leap of faith characteristic of induction'.

It has been argued, however, that both standard approaches to inductive verification and Popper's falsification approach share the same weakness – the doctrine that the truth of theories can be deduced from the ability to verify (or fail to falsify) predictions based on hypotheses (Putnam, 1971). Challenging this link (actually the symmetry tenet, prediction equals explanation, of positivism), Putnam shows that predictions are made from theories only in conjunction with 'auxiliary statements'. The auxiliary statements involve unsure assumptions about boundary or initial conditions so that false predictions cannot be regarded as falsifying a theory. The falsification approach is considered to bypass the problem of induction rather than solve it (Wulff et al., 1986).

Besides the verification issues, risk factor methods have severe limitations for uncovering multicausal mechanisms. In theory Rothman's model builds on component causes, but in practice risks are calculated for specific factors, perhaps controlling for other factors. The focus on specific factors with the corresponding neglect of complex causal processes is a fundamental weakness.

Reducing or eliminating risks will not automatically improve health or functioning (Evans, 1984; Kane et al., 1985; Kickbusch and Dean, 1992). This is because health and the influences that lead to its deterioration are multifaceted (Dubos, 1965; Juul Jensen, 1987), and accumulate over the life course (Ory et al., 1992). Many population health researchers attempt to work around these problems by combining methodological approaches with critical assessments of the research literature.

Causal Modelling in Population Health Research

Since population health research involves relationships among many complex levels and types of influences that affect health, the range of theory and methods in the researcher's repertoire is a major factor affecting the overall quality of this type of research. The social sciences provide a rich range of study designs and methodologies for research on human health and behaviour.

In quantitative population research on health, sociological methods are suitable for the investigation of wide-ranging health issues. Their great potential for population health research arises from their ability to study phenomena in contexts of occurrence. This potential depends on the theory and methods used in cohort to analyse multiple influences. Causal modelling (Simon, 1957; Abell, 1991) is the vehicle used to tap this potential. A good example of how contemporary advances in scientific methods often arise from work seeded and developed across academic disciplines,[4] causal methods used in the analysis of population data today come from a synthesis of innovations developed in econometrics, psychometrics and biometrics. Early work on causal ordering, recursive and non-recursive chains, and distinctions between endogenous and exogenous variables – all crucial developments for the options now available in causal modelling – are credited to econometricians (Bernert, 1983). Issues in causal modelling are especially relevant to the theoretical and methodological problems taken up in this book.

Methods and techniques for causal modelling, like other scientific developments, were affected by the tenets and beliefs of positivism. The historical roots of causal thinking in sociology are traced to the philosophical thinking of David Hume and Auguste Comte, and to the empirical procedures developed by John Stuart Mill for identifying causal relationships (Berk, 1991; Bernert, 1983). It was Mill (1872) that originally developed procedures for studying causes and effects in terms of necessary and sufficient conditions. Experiments were carried out to determine whether or not causal factors were invariably related to the effects of a particular cause. Mill's procedures attempted to identify causal relationships through a process of eliminating alternative explanations. Relationships identifying invariable effects of specific causes were total and absolute. Indirect, conditional and other types of relationships were not considered.

As mentioned above, the absolute and complete nature of causal relationships in this thinking could not hold up after discoveries in theoretical physics and mathematics discredited much of deterministic science by showing the fundamental limitations involved in the measurement and prediction of even the most simple physical elements. The very process of measurement, it was found, alters the measured phenomenon, introducing uncertainty into the measurement process. These discoveries firmly established stochastic methods in science.

Statistical concepts of causation had already been introduced to social scientists (Pearson, 1911). Some time before the development of quantum mechanics, Pearson had rejected absolute causation. Developing ideas of statistical association on the basis of illustrations that varying a cause of a phenomenon does not always produce the same amount of change, he introduced the idea that the less the variation in the occurrence of the phenomenon (the higher the correlation) the greater was the influence that could be ascribed to a particular cause of the phenomenon.

Pearson and his followers developed many of the statistical theories and procedures that became widely used in the analysis of data in social science investigations.[5] Still, causal analysis did not appear in sociology until the 1950s. Throughout much of the century sociology was embroiled in controversies arising both from the long-term philosophical debates about deduction and induction in science, and from divisions arising from different approaches to research in opposing schools of thought (Bernert, 1983; Abell, 1991; Bryant, 1991). Divisive traditions separating theory from empirical work and quantitative from qualitative work long prevented the type of synthesis that now appears to be occurring in the field:

> Sociologists had to believe that the alleged incommensurability between theory and research – formerly couched as deduction vs. induction – could be overcome. The first generation, for all their support of data-gathering, were theorists without method; the second generation had method but lacked theory. The next generation . . . were in search of theory more amenable to research, and methods more attuned to the state of the art. For the latter one had to look outside the discipline where the new vehicles that would make causal inquiry viable were gaining acceptability. (Bernert, 1983: 240)

From Causal Ordering to Causal Modelling

The development of causal modelling in sociology occurred essentially within the tradition of survey research. Abell traces the 'intellectual essence' for the development of causal modelling to work on the elaboration of three-variable covariation in the 1950s. The seminal work of Lazarsfeld and Rosenberg (1955) provided a framework for considering causal order in relationships among a few variables. Paul Lazarsfeld had presented an elaboration procedure in the late 1940s which provided the conceptual basis for multivariate analysis in sociology. Simon (1957; 1987), a singularly important person in the development of causal modelling, had used Lazarsfeld's elaboration formula in a set of recursive linear equations by 1954 (Bernert, 1983).

The important contributions of Rosenberg (1968) developed and systematized procedures for sorting out and elaborating complex relationships in the analysis of survey data. The very essence of this work was that relationships are not global and complete, but rather conditional, reciprocal, hidden and asymmetrical as well as symmetrical. Rosenberg's work emphasized quality and completeness in the analysis of survey data.

During the period that Lazarsfeld and Rosenberg were making their important contributions, the technological options for the analysis of relationships among multiple influences were quite limited. As theoretical advances in the natural sciences resulted in knowledge that fundamentally altered our understanding of the world and approaches to obtaining knowledge, the development of computer technology exerted a fundamental impact on research methodologies.

Multivariate modelling developed in correspondence with advances in computer technology, especially the analytic options available to researchers with the development of increasingly sophisticated software packages. Introduction of linear models (Searle, 1971) into sociological analyses opened the way for analysing multivariate problems in population health research. The concepts and techniques of causal modelling were introduced and became core elements of classical texts in the 1970s (Blalock, 1971; Duncan, 1975).

Multivariate statistical modelling is based on the view that causal relationships can be uncovered with the help of structural equations presenting sociological phenomena in algebraic form. Abell identifies major achievements arising from the introduction of causal modelling into sociological analysis: techniques were developed for studying the causal structure of any number of variables; statistical inference was made under standard assumptions; non-linear and interaction effects were introduced; measurement error, multicollinearity and other problems in causal modelling became well understood; and causal modelling became the standard approach to interpreting the validity of underlying non-observable variables.

The advantages associated with causal modelling were accompanied by problems of usage and interpretation. Cautions and controversies surrounded causal modelling from its inception. Many multivariate modelling techniques are built on assumptions that seriously limit their usefulness (Bradley, 1967; Kreiner, 1989). The major controversies, however, centre around the limitations of using partialling approaches (multivariate statistical modelling) for identifying and testing causal relationships (Berk, 1991).

Glymour and his colleagues (1987) summarize and respond to major arguments against causal modelling. The most serious issue has to do with problems of model choice due to the huge number of possible models in even low-dimensional data sets. This problem reinforced the belief of the empirical tradition in science that only experiments can contribute knowledge about causation. As in the field of epidemiology, pressure developed in sociology for using experimental designs to study causation in terms of manipulating factors for comparison in experimental and control groups (Cook and Campbell, 1979; Berk, 1991).

The Convergence of Issues

As seen in the brief overview presented above, causal thinking and methodological approaches to causal analyses in epidemiology and social survey research spring from the same philosophical roots. Similar issues have emerged in both fields. In spite of debates about empiricism and the limits of positivism, pressure grew in both fields for research approaches and methods which seek to predict the causal impact of specific factors on specific outcomes – factors separated from confounding influences by experimental design or its approximations. The principal methodological concern became to ensure that the predicted effect of the 'cause' is real and not due to some other factor(s). The purpose of random experimentation is what has been called 'context-stripping' (Guba and Lincoln, 1989), or attempts to remove the differences, variation and complexity that make up causal processes in the real world in order to observe the hypothesized effects of some particular causal factor.

The complexity of causal processes is recognized conceptually in Rothman's epidemiological model of sufficient and component causes – a model for moving beyond the deterministic thinking behind studying a cause in terms of it being a necessary and sufficient factor for predicting an effect. A recognition of complexity is also inherent in the conception and development of multivariate statistical modelling. However, in both traditions the tendency is still to focus on single causes, separating out conditioning influences. The reasons for this stem both from the focus on testing hypotheses about specific factors in empiricist science, and from the limits of widely used analytic techniques for examining complexity. Consequently, in both epidemiology and social science research on health, inconsistent and sometimes quite contradictory bodies of empirical information have been produced in research on important health issues.

Contemporary debates on problems in causal research on population health issues increasingly point to the neglect of theory (Weed, 1986; Pearce, 1990; Maclure, 1985; Abell, 1991), but as yet the tendency is towards the proliferation of research hypotheses rather than theory building. According to Popper, theories are conjectures and as such as many as possible should be subjected to empirical falsification. Preoccupation with the proliferation of 'theories' (hypotheses) has left its mark. By 1981, the so-called risk factors for coronary heart disease found in the literature had reached 240 (Hopkins and Williams, 1981); many of them are signs of symptoms of the disease processes rather than causal agents, and others are probably spurious correlations or proxy measures of complex interactions that may or may not have some contributory influence. The focus on risk factors as disease agents has become so exaggerated that the meaning of the whole exercise has been called into question, especially with regard to common degenerative diseases whose aetiology and pathophysiology are poorly understood (McCormick and Skrabanek, 1988; Ory et al., 1992).

The weaknesses of empirical prediction as an approach to expanding knowledge in population health research are tied to epistemological issues raised against positivistic science (Wulff et al., 1986; Juul Jensen, 1987). According to Pearce (1990), the scientific issues in epidemiological research arise from studying events in populations, which he sees as a barrier to the study of fundamental aetiological processes. He illustrates this with the 'theory that smoking is a cause of lung cancer'. Since smoking is a component cause of at least one sufficient cause (meaning in Rothman's model alternative combinations of components) of the disease, the theory, Pearce argues, is universal because it implies that smoking will always cause lung cancer when accompanied by the other components of one of these sufficient causes. However, since the other component causes are unknown,

> this prediction is valid only if two conditions apply. The first is that all other sufficient causes are equally distributed between smokers and nonsmokers (familiar problem of confounding). The second condition is that at least some smokers are exposed to other components of at least one sufficient cause involving smoking (the familiar problem of effect modification). (Pearce, 1990: 49)

A close examination of this explanation shows that it is not the unit of analysis (population groups versus clinical individuals) that is the fundamental problem, but rather the absence of systematic processes of theory building and empirical analyses which can elaborate interactions among influences. The smoking example illustrates the difficulty (impossibility?) of studying causation by empirically testing an array of single causes in order to predict statistical effects. The assertion that smoking is a cause of lung cancer is not a theory. The statement is a hypothesis, and testing the hypothesis in comparison groups which attempt to hold constant the moderating and mediating influences is an approach which cannot elaborate causal processes. It is an approach that unavoidably leads to a proliferation of risk factors rather than a process of building knowledge by using theory to organize and guide empirical work, and suggest new paths of inquiry.

Somewhat parallel developments occurred in sociology. Pragmatic acceptance of causal modelling based on arguments of usefulness and robustness were increasingly criticized, leading to pressures for experimental research. Berk (1991), in his overview of causal inference in sociology, reports that significant progress has been made with regard to (1) the role of chance in the occurrence of phenomena, and (2) thinking about causal effects within an experimental framework.

Pointing to discoveries in quantum mechanics and findings from research on chaos showing that predictable outcomes are undermined by minute differences in initial conditions, Berk concludes that there is widespread agreement that the social world must be viewed as stochastic. At the same time, he points to the growing emphasis on experimental research in sociology arising from the rather contradictory belief that only sociological experiments can achieve true scientific status. As in epidemiology, the high status given to experimental design resulted in increased attempts by social scientists to use randomized experiments or their approximations.

In summary, it may be concluded that while the focus and methodological conventions in epidemiology and social survey research on population health differ, a convergence with regard to underlying scientific issues developed in the two fields. In both research traditions, the view that the experimental model is the only sure approach for studying causal influences took root. Stochastic methods, developed to respond to uncertainty in causal relationships, are considered solutions for the problems of deterministic science. When statistical causal modelling is necessary, the most widely used approaches seek to estimate effects of specific causes controlling for other influences. Issues concerning inductive verification (refutation) of hypotheses about relationships between phenomena remain unresolved.

Concerns about theoretical deficits are current in both disciplines, but the theory often referred to is methodological theory – for example, theory behind statistical procedures rather than substantive theory, or theory as a separate endeavour from empirical work ('our theorists have failed us': Abell, 1991). The emphasis on experimental design and predicting statistical effects looks away from underlying mechanisms and processes of influence. It also presupposes that the future will replicate the past (Wulff et al., 1986). The contradiction inherent in the idea that the well-documented complexity known to exist in real causal forces can only be studied in experimental frameworks needs closer examination.

Major Foci of Contemporary Science

Breakthroughs in theoretical and empirical research occurring in this century are changing thinking about science, and approaches to the growth of knowledge (Crutchfield et al., 1986). Besides revealing the inadequacies of the positivistic approach to testing and verifying assertions about phenomena, fundamental discoveries in both the physical and social sciences have shifted attention to the complex interplay of forces shaping the world (May, 1976; Poston and Stewart, 1978; Khaimovich, 1992).

The rejection of beliefs in deterministic predictability arose from discoveries which discredited notions that science involves observing fixed relationships among phenomena. These discoveries, in terms of Kuhn's views, discredited the prevailing paradigm of normal science. Our growing knowledge about the fundamental complexity of causal processes, as outlined by Crutchfield and his colleagues (1986), arises from a different source: the ground breaking developments in research on dynamic systems.

In the rapidly growing interdisciplinary field of non-linear dynamics, the study of dynamic systems provides new knowledge relevant to every branch of science (Jensen, 1987; Poston and Stewart, 1978). It has long been recognized that differences in the initial conditions of a phenomenon can produce widely different outcomes. Observing or predicting outcomes based on knowledge of initial conditions to confirm causation was an aspect of attempts to revise and maintain the positivistic approach to gaining knowledge. The limitations of this view of determinism are now known. It is not only initial conditions that produce widely diverse outcomes. Research based on chaos theory has repeatedly demonstrated that small changes in the present produce much larger changes in the future at *every point* of movement in the system. 'Quantum mechanics implies that initial measurements are always uncertain, and chaos ensures that the uncertainties will quickly overwhelm the ability to make predictions' (Crutchfield et al., 1986: 41).

Recall that the symmetry condition and related tenets of positivism were developed out of a picture of the world as stable sequences of causes and effects. Given knowledge of natural laws (later revised to include approximate knowledge of initial conditions), it was believed that outcomes could be predicted within certain ranges of probability. Small deviations or influences, it was believed, could be neglected as static or random variation. Thus the focus of inquiry should be on the big effects, the global influences, the large amount of the variance explained. This view of the world is not compatible with contemporary knowledge. It has been proved that small influences and interactions among influences have profound effects on the behaviour of systems and on long-term outcomes.

Induction and confirmation continue to be important in thinking about the function of science and in empirical research, but approaches to these subjects today differ in most fields from the work of the positivists. Global induction is challenged. Recent work on observation and theory development question whether inductive confirmation has any role in obtaining general scientific knowledge (Suppe, 1977c).

It is noteworthy that in the currently more widely respected accounts of the growth of scientific knowledge, the subjects of observation and theory are central while the subjects of verification and refutation of hypotheses are generally absent. Suppe considers this to be a function of the shift in science to the active development of more sophisticated theories. Only in primitive science, he points out, where there is little concern for the development of comprehensive explanatory theories, does rejection or verification keep a central position.

The focus on verifying observations and predicting outcomes, often using statistical models based on assumptions of linearity and normal distributions, directs attention away from the small deviations, interactions and non-linear structures that compose dynamic systems. Scientists educated in linear structures and differential equations are not prepared to work with the discrete non-linear systems that are the rule rather than the exception in the biological and social sciences (May, 1976). Fine behavioural structures that actually make up systems become ignored as random 'noise'. The belief that the small effects would cancel out, that finding single important determinants would solve scientific problems and reveal the nature of reality, was the fundamental error that made justification and verifiability of empirical observations an untenable approach to expanding knowledge.

It has been found that interactions among components can lead to complex behaviour on a larger scale that cannot be deduced from knowledge of the separated parts. Crutchfield and his colleagues, pointing to the fundamental limits to our ability to make predictions, question the classical approach to verifying a theory by comparing predictions against experimental data.

It is often forgotten that experiments in themselves do not allow causal conclusions. They do not even ensure inference regarding relationships between specific factors for immediate local applicability because the context of subsequent applications may not be the same as that of the experiment (Goldstein, 1987). The fundamental problem is that contextual conditions are not a concern of inquiry in the experimental model. Glymour and his colleagues (1987) provide examples from both the physical and the social sciences of incorrect conclusions drawn from experimental studies because of failure to consider complex causal influences. Criticizing the belief that the design of experimental studies ensures the correct interpretation of the results without the need for further theoretical support, they maintain that the history of any experimental subject will show the reverse to be true.

The importance of theory in scientific work has grown in parallel with the recognition of the weaknesses of empiricism. In today's science, theory is not abstract and separated from empirical work, nor is it limited to conventional statements about how observations relate to each other. Theory involves active processes of marshalling and evaluating empirical evidence about the real world (Suppe, 1977b; Wulff et al., 1986; Juul Jensen, 1987).

Shapere's (1977) concept of theoretical domain illustrates the use of theory to organize information for purposes of discovery. Theory and observation are mutually interdependent in Shapere's thinking rather than different spheres of scientific work. Theories and theory-determined items or elements are *related* to other items in the domain of the research problem:

> scientific research is in such cases generated by items in association with one another, rather than by 'facts' in isolation from one another. Philosophers of science, working within a tradition according to which all 'facts' are 'atomic', have been blinded to this primary source of scientific problems. (p. 530).

Despite the shift of focus from prediction of statistical effects of specific factors to studying the real conditions of influence in research questions, the notion of causality has not disappeared; it has emerged as a more complex concept requiring different approaches to achieve understanding. In non-linear dynamics, 'chaos' is a technical term referring to the 'unpredictable behavior of deterministic, nonlinear systems' (Jensen, 1987). Windows of periodic behaviour are embedded in non-linear systems. Patterns emerge in dynamic systems data, focusing the scientific challenges around identifying and understanding the forces that create the patterns and those that maintain them or lead to their breakdown.

Causality in Population Health Research: Risk Factors or Dynamic Systems?

Human health is among the most complex of all dynamic systems. A growing body of research evidence points to the extreme nature of this complexity. Riley, in Chapter 2 in this volume, uses ageing to illustrate the dynamic processes shaping and preserving health or leading to decline and disease. The implications of the paradigm of age, period and cohort is that health at any given time integrates the long-term influences arising from being born into and growing up in a particular historical context along with the contemporary influences of the social and physical environment. This means that accumulated effects and current influences constantly interact in all people, in the apparently healthy as well as in the acutely ill or in chronically diseased persons. Since most people are not clinically infected most of the time, in spite of exposure to disease producing organisms regularly present in the human body and the physical environment, it is not possible to understand infection by concentrating on the prevalence and toxicity of specific germs. The occurrence of infection is a less important subject of inquiry than understanding the processes involved in moving from exposure to overt symptoms and disease (Dubos, 1965).

The same logic readily applies to chronic disease processes and to health maintenance. This is illustrated by the proliferation of contradictory findings for a multitude of disease risks without any explanation of processes of occurrence. The key to understanding these causal processes is clearly the ability to elaborate and understand complexity. The interacting systems involved will always overwhelm predictions of 'independent effects' of any single factor, reducing them to very limited and uncertain information.

Wulff and his colleagues (1986), discussing weaknesses in empiricist thinking, illustrate that causes of a specific outcome are usually neither necessary nor sufficient, but rather 'nonredundant components of an effective causal complex'. The selection of any single cause, they maintain, reflects the interests of the person who makes the choice. Illustrating their conclusions with examples from health research, they point out that, for example, the cause of alcoholism, depending on the definer, reflects the total range of norms, interests and political beliefs in society.

The emerging debates on AIDS research provide a contemporary example of persistent dominant focus on a germ, the HIV virus, in spite of evidence suggesting the need to learn more about host conditions and concurrent disease processes (Root-Berstein, 1992). An example in research on ageing is the persistent focus on osteoporosis as a female disease related to menopause, in spite of evidence pointing to lifestyle influences escalating this ageing process in both men and women (Anderson, 1992).

Evidence of the importance of multilevel causal interactions is seen as the fact that physical, social and behavioural influences are associated with a wide range of outcomes rather than specific diseases (Ory et al., 1992). One of the fastest growing bodies of knowledge comes from research on relationships among psychosocial factors and physiochemical processes (Vogt, 1992; Pelletier, 1992). In research focused on complex forces shaping health, new knowledge is being obtained by elaborating interactions and pathways of influence (Ory et al., 1992; Dean, 1986; 1992).

Given the growing body of knowledge about multilevel interactions and pathways, a question which naturally arises is why so much of population health research continues to focus on specific factors. It would appear that continued adherence to experimental design as the ultimate and only sure way to study causation, and to the emphasis on predicting 'independent' effects of specific factors rather than elaborating the contextual nature of causal influences, is at least part of the explanation for the neglect of more dynamic approaches to population health research.

Disease processes involved in cancer, coronary disease and other of the more serious health conditions in developed countries often exist as non-fatal and non-detected pathological deviations (Goldman et al., 1983; McFarlane et al., 1987). Any suspected aetiological agent that is associated with increased use of diagnostic technology will also be associated with increased detection of disease, with the result that the apparent increase in occurrence of a disease will be attributed to some agent rather than the detection process (Feinstein, 1988) and the concurrent causal influences.

Attempts to remove these problems by experimental design are generally not feasible in investigations of complex multicausal influences. Even if feasible they would be unethical in most cases. Stratification analyses quickly became overwhelmed by the complex range of 'confounding' influences, leaving the researcher with multivariate statistical modelling which has been considered the less desirable approach in some research circles. A far more fundamental problem is, however, the inability to assess the complex meaning of these silent disease processes. How did they develop? Over how long a period? Why do they differ in similar groups of people with the same exposure? Why do many people live normally with a dangerous disease until they die from other diseases or accidents, while some people die of the disease?

Applying contemporary scientific thinking to population health research points to neglected aspects of our origins, to the epidemiological triad of environment, host and agent (Duncan, 1988; Lilienfeld and Lilienfeld, 1980; Fox et al., 1970), to the elaboration of conditional relationships in survey research (Rosenberg, 1968). It also suggests that rather than shunning multivariate causal modelling because of problems in model selection, we need newer approaches focused on complexity. Disease agents can only be understood in terms of the interacting processes that determine the impact of specific factors. This applies to variables influencing behaviours, treatments, use of professional services and effectiveness of services as well as to those affecting health more directly.

Theory to Elaborate Complexity

The contemporary alternative to radical empiricism is a concern for understanding causal processes in the contexts in which they occur in the real world. Shapere's notion of scientific domains as the pathways through which scientific knowledge accumulates reflects this shift towards problem solving in the context of real situations involving moderating and conditional influences rather than predicting probable outcomes of specific hypothesized factors. Domains, in this thinking, are composed of elements which, taken together, form bodies of information.

The idea of a theoretical domain recognizes the importance of relationships among entities rather than their reduction. Problem solving has to do with the relationships among elements or components of the domain, a notion where theory interfaces with empirical elaboration of conditions of influence in contrast to the prediction of global truths. Observation and theory become *mutually interdependent*, rather than being separate and distinct types of scientific endeavour: 'what was, at a certain stage of science, a "theory" answering a problem about a domain can, at a later stage, itself become a domain (or, more usually, a part of a domain) to be investigated and accounted for' (Shapere, 1977: 529).

Applied to research on population health, theoretical domains may be thought of as developmental frameworks for elaborating causal processes to build bodies of knowledge in substantive areas. The complexity of the dynamic systems involved in health issues constitutes a challenge, but work on complexity in many areas of scientific inquiry suggests that the barriers are not insurmountable. There are examples of theoretical domains where much has already been achieved. As mentioned above, host susceptibility is a theoretical framework for more holistic approaches to research that focuses on human health rather than on specific diseases. Strong evidence exists in support of this theory. It is known that the general decline in incidence, prevalence and mortality from infectious diseases that has occurred in industrialized countries is due to improvements in population host resistance to different diseases (Dubos, 1965; McKeown, 1976).

Other important theoretical domains are social stratification, social support, coping and lifestyle. Besides the age, period and cohort paradigm taken up by Riley and Wolinsky, work needs to progress on the biopsychosocial model also discussed by Riley in Chapter 2. She points to the errors that accrued from atheoretical empirical studies and shows us that the different types of research designs and analytic approaches all have strengths and weaknesses for building bodies of scientific information. The role of theory is not limited to stimulating research questions and informing design: it also serves to alert us to misinterpretations and fallacies. This entails a process whereby theory guides empirical work, the results of which feed back into the confirmation and modification of theory, and whereby, as suggested by Shapere, a theory or empirical results derived from a theory may lead to a new problem domain. In this way a theory could address Pearce's (1990) ideal of 'laying out the fundamental processes underlying a given set of phenomena'.

Methods to Inform Theory

While the neglect of theory is increasingly recognized as a problem, less attention has been given to the role of methods in the development and testing of theory. When inappropriate methods are used in an investigation, or suitable methods are not available, the methodological problems which arise interfere with theory assessment and modification. Wolinsky, in Chapter 3, identifies the limitations of methods that have been used to study age, period and cohort differences, and points to problems of statistical confounding and interactions among variables. Here again deficits in theory building are recognized as a serious problem.

Similarly, the pressure for experimental research on health questions diverts attention away from developing approaches to causal modelling which integrate theory building and modification with the use of multivariate statistical techniques in a manner that builds on their advantages for elaborating complex relationships, while at the same time addressing problems of model selection and interpretation of findings.

Model selection in causal analysis is only one of many areas in scientific and professional work requiring decision making strategies. Faust (1984), documenting extensively the cognitive limits of human judgement in scientific and clinical work, outlines approaches for dealing with these limitations in research on complex problems. According to Faust, theory evaluation and discovery are fundamental aspects of guiding scientific work in the face of human cognitive limitations. He also points to the importance of scientific collaboration, especially interdisciplinary collaboration among scientists working on difficult problems, as an essential aspect of transcending cognitive limitations. The third approach outlined by Faust involves developing methods for handling data in ways that reduce the information processing load. This means developing systems for representing and analysing data that incorporate decision making rules that allow more information to be processed simultaneously.

A major problem in population health research has been that even when theory is multicausal, the research design and statistical analysis often test single causes. Cox, in Chapter 7, contrasting empirical and substantive statistical models, illustrates the dangers of empirical models that are not guided by knowledge of the subject of the analysis. The choice of statistical methods, he points out, must match the complexity of the research problem. The methods used to study causal processes must be capable of elaborating complexity and contributing to theory modification and development. The models presented by Whittaker, Wermuth and Arminger in Chapters 8–10 provide methodological options for elaborating antecendent, intervening and hidden relationships in analyses that examine numerous variables simultaneously, thus moving beyond the constraints faced by Lazarsfeld and Rosenberg in their work on the elaboration of three-variable covariation.

These techniques, however, cannot become a basis for scientific causal modelling unless theory is used to guide an interplay of available substantive knowledge and model choice in the elaboration of relationships among multiple influences. This involves using the empirical findings to build and strengthen the theory. Vague theories provide predictions no matter what the truth really is, and decisions guided only by statistical significance are not scientific (Maclure, 1985). Refutation of a null hypothesis only suggests that an association exists under the conditions present in a given table. Its meaning depends on moderating and conditioning influences.

Considerable advances have already been made in options for integrating theory and methods to elaborate causal processes within theoretical domains. Many of these options are discussed in the chapters that follow. Work in a theoretical domain involves investigating all types of scientific issues within the domain. This means that the research design, data collection and measurement issues discussed by Nesselroade and Hershberger, McQueen and Kreiner respectively are fundamental aspects of the problem solving work. Intraindividual variability and variable stability are important scientific issues. In elaboration, it must be emphasized, no single design or analytic technique suffices. Thus elaboration involves multimethod approaches to scientific questions. It should be mentioned in this regard that the importance of retrospective research should be reinstated. The discrediting of retrospective investigations in some circles came from the undue faith placed in prediction, a faith overlooking that prediction is a mere description of a temporal relation to an event rather than an explanation.[6]

In closing, the importance of qualitative and indirect evidence, subjects generally not taken up in this book, should be recognized. Scriven (1962), illustrating that there is no difference between direct and indirect evidence in establishing a scientific conclusion, shows that explanations can be supported by evidence about 'qualitative necessary conditions whereas even a conditional prediction requires quantitative sufficient conditions'. This fact, he points out, is lost when researchers proceed on the basis of the common assumption that causes are simply sufficient conditions. Since exact quantitative sufficient conditions recur rarely, if ever, causal statements based on predictions are what Scriven calls dubious determinism rather than even genuine conditional predictions:

> The problem of direct vs. indirect confirmation which arises here is of great importance throughout structural logic. To say that 'same cause, same effect' is a determinist's slogan is not to say it has no empirical content. It has, and it is actually false . . . What it lacks is a single-case applicability and hence direct confirmability when complex systems are involved – for it is often impossible to specify what counts as the 'same conditions'. (p.189)

The discrediting of positivistic science, especially notions that prediction is comparable to explanation, led some to the incorrect conclusion that a realistic perspective in science precludes the study of statistical relationships in variable-centred analyses. Statistical analyses of population data can focus on direct and indirect connections among influences rather than predictions. Indirect relationships are components of causal processes, and thus important to identify in causal modelling (Ory et al., 1992; Dean, 1992). As Scriven points out, understanding is gained by any process that locates a puzzling phenomenon in a system of relationships. The great potential of the analytic methods discussed in this book arises from exactly that quality.

Notes

The author respectfully acknowledges the comments and criticisms made on an earlier version of this chapter by Theodor Litman, Mike Finch, Jørgen Hilden, Henrik Wulff and David McQueen.

1 Logical positivism, developed in the twentieth century, is a form of empiricism building on logical analysis, in contrast to the historical analysis which formed the basis of the original doctrine of positivism developed by Auguste Comte in the

nineteenth century (Barrett, 1962). As such logical positivism was influenced more by the empiricism of David Hume, and the later work of Bertrand Russell and Alfred North Whitehead on mathematical logic, than by Comte's historical postivism. While these intellectual roots exerted fundamental influence on the later development of logical positivism, it originated as a Germanic movement growing out of the doctrine of mechanistic materialism which combined views from Comptean positivism with materialism and mechanism (Suppe, 1977a).

The doctrine of mechanistic materialism held that all existence is governed by mechanical laws inherent in things themselves. Matter was considered primary and independent of individual perception. Thus knowledge about the mechanistic laws governing life was to be obtained by a scientific method of empirical observation without *a priori* speculation. Challenges to this doctrine led to three competing schools of thought: mechanistic materialism, a form of neo-Kantianism, and a neo-positivism developed by Mach. A version of the latter, especially a focus on verifiability in scientific work, was adopted in the 1920s and 1930s by the Vienna Circle. Organized around Rudolf Carnap and Moritz Schlick, the members of the Vienna Circle included a large proportion of mathematicians and physicists, which explains the influence of mathematical logic on the movement.

2 The concepts of necessary cause and sufficient cause, first used in the scientific procedures developed by John Stuart Mill, have been central to both challenges to empiricist science and attempts to modify and reform its weaknesses. In addition to later references made in this chapter, see e.g. Wulff et al. (1986) and Rothman (1986).

3 Multivariate analysis is used in epidemiology, but as a less preferable alternative when stratification, the 'first-line method for controlling confounding and evaluating effect modification', is unmanageable (Rothman, 1986: 306). The major concern with regard to multivariate statistical modelling is that it is considered inferior to stratification analysis for the purposes of causal inference.

4 This has probably always been the case within the constraints of less rapid dissemination of information in earlier times, and therefore slower cross-fertilization of ideas among innovators.

5 This unavoidably shallow overview neglects many important developments and innovators. The significance of the seminal work of Sewall Wright in the 1930s on path coefficients for methods discussed in this book should, however, be noted.

6 The 'retrodictions' and 'postdictions' long used in the work of archaeologists, geologists and many other fields, including much good work in the social sciences, have the same logical structure as predictions. 'Predictions and postdictions can be obtained from arguments of virtually any logical form' (Scriven, 1962) and, as discussed above, 'initial conditions' will always be overwhelmed by complex non-linear causal structures.

References

Abell, Peter (1991) 'Methodological achievements in sociology over the past few decades with special reference to the interplay of quantitative and qualitative methods', in Christopher G. A. Bryant and Henk A. Becker (eds), *What Has Sociology Achieved?* New York: Macmillan.

Anderson, David (1992) 'Osteoporosis in men', *British Medical Journal*, 305: 489–490.

Barrett, William (1962) 'Introduction to Part Three: Positivism' in W. Barrett and H.D. Aiken (eds), *Philosophy in the Twentieth Century*, vol. 3. New York: Random House.

Berk, Richard A. (1991) 'Causal inference for sociological data', in N.J. Smelser (ed.), *Handbook of Sociology*. Newbury Park, CA: Sage. pp. 155–72.

Bernert, Christopher (1983) 'The career of causal analysis in American sociology', *The British Journal of Sociology*, 34(2): 230–54.

Blalock, Hubert M. Jr (1971) Causal Models in the Social Sciences. Chicago: Aldine-Atherton.

Bohr, N. (1934) *Atomic Theory and the Description of Nature*. Cambridge: Cambridge University Press.

Bradley, James V. (1967) *Distribution-Free Statistical Tests*. Englewood Cliffs, NJ: Prentice-Hall.

Bromberger, S. (1966) 'Why questions', in R. Colodny (ed.), *Mind and Cosmos: Exploration in the Philosophy of Science*. Pittsburgh, PA: University of Pittsburgh Press.

Bryant, Christopher G.A. (1991) 'Tales of innocence and experience: developments in sociological theory since 1950', in Christopher G.A. Bryant and Henk A. Becker (ed), *What Has Sociology Achieved?* New York: Macmillan.

Cook, Thomas D. and Campbell, Donald T. (1979) *Quasiexperimentation*. Chicago: Rand McNally.

Crutchfield, James P., Farmer, J. Doyne, Packard, Norman H. and Shaw, Robert S. (1986) 'Chaos', *Scientific American*, December: 46–57.

Dean, Kathryn (1986) 'Social support and health: pathways of influence', *Journal of Health Promotion*, 1: 133–50.

Dean, Kathryn (1992) 'Health-related behavior: concepts and methods', in Marcia G. Ory, Ronald P. Abeles and Paula Darby Lipman (eds), *Aging, Health and Behavior*. Newbury Park, CA: Sage. pp. 27–66.

Dubos, R. (1965) *Man Adapting*. New Haven, CT: Yale University Press. pp. 164–5.

Duncan, David F. (1988). *Epidemiology*. New York: Macmillan.

Duncan, Dudley (1975) *Introduction to Structural Equation Models*. New York: Academic Press.

Evans, J.G. (1984) 'Prevention of age-associated loss of autonomy: epidemiological approaches', *Journal of Chronic Diseases*, 37: 353–63.

Faust, D. (1984) *The Limits of Scientific Reasoning*. Minneapolis: Unversity of Minnesota Press.

Feinstein, Alvan R. (1988) 'Scientific standards in epidemiologic studies of the menace of daily life', *Science*, 242: 1257–63.

Fox, John P., Hall, Carrie and Elveback, Lila (1970) *Epidemiology: Man and Disease*. London: Macmillan.

Glymour, R., Scheines, R., Spirtes, P. and Kelly, K. (1987) *Discovering Causal Structure: Artificial Intelligence, Philosophy of Science and Statistical Modelling*. New York: Academic Press.

Goldman, L., Sayson, R., Robbins, S., Cohn, L., Bettmann, M. and Weisberg, M. 'The value of the autopsy in three medical eras', (1983) *New England Journal of Medicine*, 308: 1000–5.

Goldstein, H. (1987) *Multilevel Models in Educational and Social Research*. London: Oxford University Press.

Guba, G. and Lincoln, Y.S. (1989) *Fourth Generation Evaluation*. Newbury Park, CA: Sage.

Heisenberg, W. (1958) *Physics and Philosophy: the Revolution in Philosophy*. New York: Harper.
Hempel, C. and Oppenheim, P. (1948) 'Studies in the logic of explanation', *Philosophy of Science*, 15: 135–75.
Hopkins, P.N. and Williams, R.R. (1981) 'A survey of 246 suggested coronary risk factors', *Atherosclerosis*, 40: 1–52.
Jensen, Roderick V. (1987) 'Classical chaos', *American Scientist*, 75: 168–81.
Juul Jensen, U. (1987) *Practice and Progress: a Theory for the Modern Health-Care System*. Oxford: Blackwell Scientific.
Kane, R.L., Kane, R. and Arnold, A. (1985) 'Prevention in the elderly: risk factors', *Health Services Research*. 19: 945–1006.
Khaimovich, L. (1992) 'Recent developments in nonlinear dynamics: unfolding the meaning of sociologically relevant concepts'. Paper prepared for the 1992 American Statistical Association meeting.
Kickbusch, I. and Dean, K. (1992) 'Research for health: challenge of the nineties', in Shunichi Araki (ed.), *Behavioral Medicine: an Integrated Biobehavioral Approach to Health and Illness*. Amsterdam: Elsevier. pp. 299–307.
Kreiner, S. (1989) 'Statistical analysis of complex health and social data', *Social Science and Medicine*, 29 (2): 253–8.
Kuhn, T.S. (1962) *The Structure of Scientific Revolutions*, 2nd edn. Chicago: University of Chicago Press.
Lazarsfeld, P.F. and Rosenberg, M. (1955) *The Language of Social Research*. Glencoe, IL: Free Press.
Lilienfeld, A.M. and Lilienfeld, D.E. (1980) *Foundations of Epidemiology*. New York: Oxford University Press.
Maclure, Malcolm (1985) 'Popperian refutation in epidemiology', *American Journal of Epidemiology*, 121: 343–50.
May, R. (1976) 'Simple mathematical models with very complicated dynamics', *Nature*, 261: 459–67.
McCormick, J. and Skrabanck, P. (1988) 'Coronary heart disease is not preventable by population interventions', *The Lancet*, 8615: 839.
McFarlane, M.J., Feinstein, A.R., Wells, C.K. and Chan, C.K. (1987) *Journal of the American Medical Association*, 258: 331.
McKeown, T. (1976) *The Modern Rise of Population*. New York: Academic Press.
Miettinen, Olli S. (1985) *Theoretical Epidemiology*. New York: Wiley.
Mill, J. Stuart (1872) *A System of Logic*. London: Longmans, Green, Reader and Dyer.
Ory, Marcia G., Abeles, Ronald P. and Lipman, Paul Darby (eds) (1992) *Aging, Health, and Behavior*. Newbury Park, CA: Sage.
Pais, A. (1991) *Niels Bohr's Times in Physics, Philosophy and Policy*, Oxford: Clarendon Press.
Pearce, Neil (1990) 'White swans, black ravens, and lame ducks: necessary and sufficient causes in epidemiology', *Epidemiology*, 1: 47–50.
Pearson, K. (1911) *The Grammar of Science*, 3rd edn. London: A. and C. Black
Pelletier, Kenneth R. (1992) 'Mind–body health: research, clinical, and policy applications', *American Journal of Health Promotion*, 6: 345–58.
Popper, K.R. (1965) *The Logic of Scientific Discovery*. New York: Harper and Row.
Poston, T. and Stewart, I. (1978) *Catastrophe Theory and its Applications*. Belmont, CA: Fearon-Pitman.

Putnam, Hilary (1971) 'On the "corroboration" of theories', in P. Schlipp (ed.), *The Philosophy of Karl R. Popper*. LaSalle, IL: Open Court.
Quine, W.V. (1962) 'Two dogmas of empiricism', in W. Barrett and H.D. Aiken (eds), *Philosophy in the Twentieth Century*, vol. 3. New York: Random House.
Root-Berstein, R.S. (1992) 'AIDS is more than HIV', *Genetic Engineering News*, 12 (13): 4–7.
Rosen, George (1958) *A History of Public Health*. New York: MD.
Rosenberg, M. (1968) *The Logic of Survey Analysis*. New York: Basic Books.
Rothman, Kenneth J. (1986) *Modern Epidemiology*. Boston: Little Brown.
Schaffner, K. (1969) 'Correspondence rules', *Philosophy of Science*, 36: 280–90.
Scriven, M. (1962) 'Explanations, predictions, and laws', in H. Feigl and G. Maxwell (eds), *Minnesota Studies in the Philosophy of Science*. Minneapolis: University of Minnesota Press.
Searle, S. (1971) *Linear Models*. New York: Wiley.
Shapere, D. (1964) 'The structure of scientific revolutions', *Philosophical Review*, 73: 383–94.
Shapere, D. (1977) 'Scientific theories and their domains', in Frederik Suppe (ed.), *The Structure of Scientific Theories*. Chicago: University of Illinois Press.
Simon, H. (1957) *Models of Man: Social and Rational*. New York: Wiley.
Simon, H. (1987) 'Foreword', in R. Glymour, R. Scheines, P. Spirtes and K. Kelly (eds), *Discovering Causal Structure*. New York: Academic Press.
Sparling, P.F. (1983) 'Bacterial virulence and pathogenesis: an overview', *Review of Infectious Diseases*, 5: S637–46.
Suppe, Frederik (1977a) 'The search for philosophic understanding of scientific theories', in Frederik Suppe (ed.), *The Structure of Scientific Theories*. Chicago: University of Illinois Press.
Suppe, Frederik (1977b) 'Hilary Putnam's "Scientific explanation" ', in Frederik Suppe (ed.), *The Structure of Scientific Theories*. Chicago: University of Illinois Press. pp. 424–33.
Suppe, Frederik (1977c) 'Afterword', in Frederik Suppe (ed.), *The Structure of Scientific Theories*. Chicago: University of Illinois Press. pp. 617–729.
Toulmin, S. (1961) *Foresight and Understanding*. New York: Harper and Row.
Vogt, Thomas M. (1992) 'Aging, stress, and illness: psychobiological linkages', in Marcia G. Ory, Ronald P. Abeles and Paula Darby Lipman (eds), *Aging, Health, and Behavior*. Newbury Park, CA: Sage. pp. 207–36.
Weed, Douglas L. (1986) 'On the logic of causal inference', *American Journal of Epidemiology*, 123: 965–78.
Wilson, F. (1967) 'Explanation in Aristotle, Newton and Toulmin', *Philosophy of Science*, 34: 291–310.
Wulff, H., Pedersen, S. and Rosenberg, R. (1986) *Philosophy of Medicine*, Oxford: Blackwell Scientific .

2

A Theoretical Basis for Research on Health

Matilda White Riley

Introduction

This chapter outlines a broad theoretical framework for research on the multiple influences affecting health in populations. These influences, and their antecedents and consequences, reach far beyond conventional studies of individual characteristics and behaviours. They rest instead on theories involving people's entire lives – from genetic makeup and family background to diverse life-course experiences; they rest also on the complex interplay between individual lives and the changing social environment.

Among the numerous theories relevant for particular research objectives, this chapter outlines one transcendent multidisciplinary theory. This theory seems especially appropriate as a guide to research on the varied processes producing states of health or disease in populations, and to past and potential future changes in these states. The theory is dynamic. It involves two universal processes underlying more specific propositions about influences on health: (1) ageing and (2) the succession of cohorts. The population is continually being composed and recomposed by the succession of birth cohorts, as new members enter the society, grow older from birth to death, and ultimately die or move away. The factors producing health or disease are inherent in the interplay between the successive cohorts of people who are growing older and the social and cultural changes in the environing society.

Central to this theory are two radical principles that hold enormous implications for understanding health and for designing research to guide interventions that can improve it. First, the process of ageing from birth to death is *not* immutable or fixed for all time, but changes across and within cohorts as society changes. Secondly, the older people of the future will *not* be the same as the older people of today; they belong to *cohorts* who were born at different times and have undergone different experiences.

In this chapter, the theory is outlined as a conceptual model or paradigm, that is an organizing image or set of ideas about the nature of the phenomena under scrutiny (see Riley, 1963: Unit 1).[1]

Use of the paradigm is illustrated through four interrelated theoretical approaches for designing and interpreting research on influences affecting health. These approaches, derived from the broad conceptual framework, are designed to be translated into empirical research operations. They identify, for particular research objectives, what questions are to be asked, what influences are to be examined, and how empirical procedures are to be used as tools in finding answers to these questions. Varied examples of health-related research, utilizing a wide range of methods, illustrate the use of each of the theoretical approaches. These examples suggest how, through such approaches, theory can be used to broaden understanding of specific findings, guard against fallacious interpretation, and identify substantive clues and insights about health-related processes that require still further specification and testing.

Problems and Fallacies in Atheoretical Research

Our early experiences in developing the theory described here are instructive: they demonstrate that lack of adequate theory can cause serious misinterpretation of empirical findings. These experiences relate broadly to a theory of age, comprising particular foci on health and many other aspects of human lives, populations and societies. Indeed, the conceptual model used in this chapter is called the 'paradigm for analysis of age', since the processes of ageing and cohort succession, and their impact on changes in the population, are all linked to age.

Those early experiences emphasized the fact that, despite the extraordinary power of age as an empirical variable, most studies were shockingly atheoretical. Two decades ago, when a number of us prepared an inventory of findings on the middle and later years (Riley and Foner, 1968), we came upon such puzzling statements as these:

1 Intelligence peaks among young people in their late teens, and then declines with age.
2 For many physiological functions, the age curves show steady decreases from age 30 to age 60 (as in nerve conduction velocity, maximum breathing capacity, blood glucose levels while fasting: the classic findings by Nathan Shock, 1976).

But what did these findings mean? Did they really mean (as they were widely interpreted to mean) that people, because they age, inevitably lose their ability to think or remember or function effectively? We didn't think so. But at that time there was no theory to help in finding answers.

To approach the dilemma, we invented a seemingly absurd example. The finding: in the United States older people had completed fewer grades in school than had middle-aged or younger people. The absurd interpretation: that the number of school grades they had actually attended had dropped *because they grew older*? Here the fallacy became obvious. Older people did indeed differ in educational level from young people, but the explanation of the difference could *not* be found in the *process of ageing*. In this instance, the differences clearly arose because social change affected the amounts of schooling offered to *different cohorts* at different periods in the past. Yet we found numerous instances of such fallacious interpretations – and they persist to this day – buttressing the dangerous stereotype of 'inevitable ageing decline', and in particular confounding understandings of the risks and the setting affecting health (Riley, 1981).

Such alarming experiences literally goaded us into the search for theories that could prevent fallacious interpretations and faulty research designs further confounding theoretical understandings. We gave the name 'life-course fallacy' to the erroneous assumption (as in the above examples) that cross-sectional age differences refer exclusively to the process of ageing – without regard for the cohort differences that may also be implicated (Riley, 1973). And we began several years of work on a conceptual model, illustrated here in the paradigm for analysis of age. This conceptual model aims to explain the complex power of age as an empirical variable, and to guide the design of appropriate research for examining and interpreting it (Riley et al., 1972).

Paradigm for Analysis of Age

This paradigm (now well known to students of the sociology of age, and similar in form to the Lexis diagram used by demographers) is schematized in Figure 2.1. This is a space bounded on its vertical axis by years of age (from 0 to 100 or more), and on its horizontal axis by historical time. I will quickly identify four major conceptual elements, before considering in further detail how each relates to influences on health. First, each diagonal bar represents a cohort of people (all born during the same period) who are ageing from birth to death – moving across time and upward with age. As they age, they are changing socially and psychologically as well as biologically; moving through roles; accumulating knowledge, attitudes and experiences. In the meantime, secondly, there is an entire series of diagonal bars, that is successive cohorts of people are continually being born, passing through different historical periods, dying, and

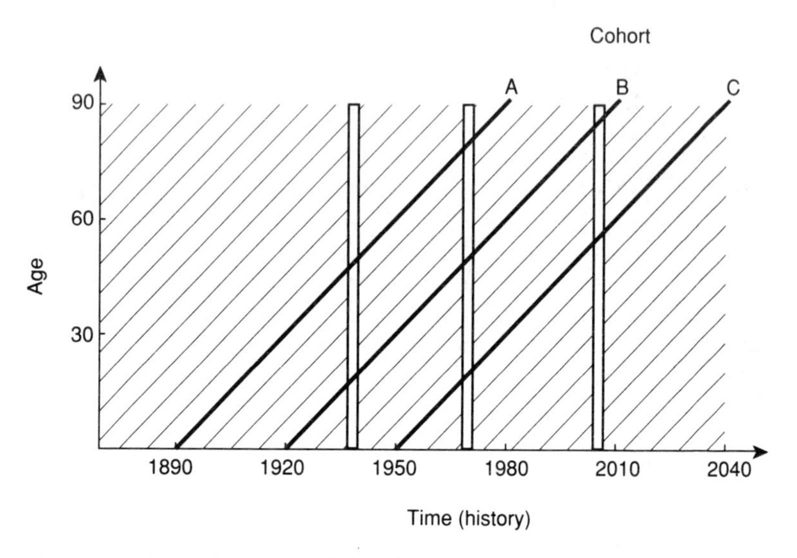

Figure 2.1 *Paradigm for analysis of age*

being replaced by new cohorts. Thirdly, at any single moment of history, a cross-section slice cuts through the successive cohorts (as shown for 1980) and divides people into age strata, from the youngest to the oldest, all of whom coexist and interact with one another.[2] Fourthly, over time, as society moves through historical events and changes, this vertical slice moves across the space from one date to the next. And you can begin to see how the people in particular age strata are no longer the same people; they have been replaced by younger entrants from more recent cohorts with more recent life experiences.

These four complex elements can be used as guides to four corresponding conceptual approaches to empirical work on particular aspects of health, its antecendents and consequences, and its changes. Since the focus in this book is on health in populations, I will begin with the cross-section approach, then proceed with the life-course approach, the cohort approach and the social change approach (see Riley et al., 1988; Riley, 1987), along the way noting some complementary conceptual perspectives.

The Cross-Section Approach

The cross-section approach – the familiar view of people of all ages in the population at a single time (corresponding to one perpendicular line in Figure 2.1, as in 1980) – is essential for understanding patterns of health in the population. It is the theoretical basis for various multifactional research designs that describe and compare the health of older and younger people at a given time, and that describe current relationships among people with age-related differences in health. Numerous examples of such studies are well known. Thus, age differences are important in understanding the prevalence of diseases. Many chronic diseases are most prevalent among the increasing numbers of older people, raising significant questions about antecedents and consequences. Even AIDS, though thought from clinical experience to be a young person's disease, appears in cross-section at every age; it even afflicts persons in their 50s and 60s, thereby pointing to neglected population segments that require special attention.

Cross-section views of people in the several age strata are also important for understanding the societal context affecting health and illness. For example, because of current social pressures on older people to withdraw from work, some have come to define themselves as incompetent, have allowed their skills to atrophy, and sometimes have become mentally or physically ill. Particular studies show how age can operate with detriment to health, as health care providers often spend less time with older than with younger patients, and give them more palliative than interventionist treatments; or how doctor–patient relationships differ with the age of the patient, with older patients being more deferential and less independent in decision making than younger ones. Issues of intergenerational equity arise in the United States, as a larger share of the federal budget is reportedly spent on the health needs of older people than on the needs of children.

Thus the theory of an age-stratified population points to epidemiological issues of the nature and causes of prevalence of health or disease; and in turn the findings from cross-section studies can feed back into the theory. Useful as this cross-section approach is, however, if we want to understand the dynamic processes through which age affects health and its consequences, the three other approaches are essential.

The Life-Course Approach

The life-course approach traces over time the lives of members of a single cohort in order to examine health, and its antecendents and consequences, as related to the ageing process (see one of the diagonal lines, such as cohort A, in Figure 2.1). Here, theories of the life course are often translated into multifactional longitudinal or panel analyses. This approach has been used in many studies to isolate early-life risk factors for subsequent heart disease; or to demonstrate that, even in late life, prevention, such as stopping cigarette smoking, is followed by reduced subsequent rates of morbidity (cf. Kaplan and Haan, 1989); or to show how the course of protracted disease, such as cancer, interacts with concurrent processes of psychosocial and biological ageing (Riley, 1983).

The life-course approach cannot demonstrate causality, but it can contribute importantly to causal analysis by establishing the time order of correlated variables. For example, a crucial question in modern societies is why reported ill health is so widely correlated with early retirement. There are indications that these reports are often mere *ex post facto* rationalizations of people's dissatisfaction with work. However, the alternative explanation has also obtained support from the longitudinal finding that reports of ill health often *precede* the decision to retire. Thus the life-course approach can help to distinguish among types of individuals for whom health operates differentially as a factor in the retirement process.

However, this approach is also vulnerable to its own type of conceptual misinterpretation – to the fallacy I call 'cohort centrism'. This is the fallacy of erroneously assuming that members of all cohorts will age in exactly the same fashion as members of the cohort under study. In fact, different cohorts, responding to different periods of history, can age in different ways with different implications for health. Thus the somewhat puzzling finding[3] of *lowered* mortality rates in certain cohorts who had experienced World War II contrasts with the finding of *high* mortality rates in the more recent cohorts. Scrutiny of these cohort differences in mortality points to the dramatic changes in cholesterol consumption involved: the wartime shortages of meat and dairy products that had protected the earlier cohorts were replaced for the post-war cohorts by the availability of such foods and the return to high-cholesterol diets. Thus to have assumed that the dietary patterns observed in the earlier cohorts would persist for all subsequent cohorts would have constituted a fallacy. Only through comparison with the more recent cohorts does the explanation emerge, as the conceptual scheme reminds us.

The Cohort Approach

Still more powerful, then, than the life-course approach, with its focus on the lives of members of a single cohort, is the cohort[4] approach. This approach focuses on health over the lives of members of two or more successive cohorts (comparing a series of diagonals in Figure 2.1). As you will note, each diagonal spans a unique period of history (on the horizontal axis). Here the theory has the special property of requiring simultaneous examination of life-course patterns of health or disease and also of cohort differences in these patterns – as age-related health processes may be influenced by social change. Thus the approach helps to conceptualize the complicated relationships between ageing and cohort succession. It avoids cohort centrism. And it adds in several significant ways to understanding life-course influences on health. I will list a few.

First, the theoretical principle that the ageing process is variable can be examined in relation to the multiple influences on health. The conditions under which age-related influences on health are mutable can be probed by comparing cohorts of individuals who grow old under particular historical or future conditions. Thus, it has been clearly demonstrated that members of cohorts already old differ markedly from those in cohorts not yet old in many critical respects that can influence health: diet, exercise, standard of living, education, work history, medical care, and experience with acute versus chronic diseases. Such findings have pointed to possible linkages with social changes affecting health over historical time – as in standard of living, scientific knowledge, public health measures or popular beliefs. Research designs examining cohort influences on individual life-course patterns of health often treat cohort membership as a contextual characteristic of individuals, to be analysed in conjunction with gender, education and other individual characteristics.

Cohort comparisons alert us, in the second place, to the distinction between age-relevant and *age-irrelevant* influences on health. A prime example of age irrelevancy is a nation-wide epidemic, such as the influenza epidemic of 1917–18, which cuts across all ages in the population at a single period and hence can be understood in terms not of life-course patterns but of conditions characterizing that particular historical period. In contrast, the classic analysis by Frost (1939) emphasized age relevance. Frost was able to explain the changing death rates from tuberculosis only by demonstrating the same persistent relationship to age in a whole series of cohorts, regardless of period. By identifying these age-relevant life-course patterns, Frost was able to find support for his postulated theories about the vulnerabilities and aetiologies of the disease (as related to primary infection in early life and the once fatal secondary form of the disease among adults: see the important discussion by Susser, 1969; also Riley et al., 1972: 50–1). Thus, by starting with a theory of cohort differences, Frost could use his data to feed back into a theory of disease.

Though such period events as epidemics, wars or depressions may sometimes prove age irrelevant at the population level (when members of each cohort are aggregated), other analyses examine how these events affect the ageing process differentially as they impinge on individuals within the coexisting cohorts of persons who differ in age. For example, the Great Depression was found to have more traumatic consequences for the future lives of boys in cohorts who were younger at the time of the event than for the lives of boys in earlier cohorts who were older, and these consequences were further affected by the economic status of the individual boys (Elder and Rockwell, 1979). Again, a theory led to a new order of substantive understanding.

Thirdly, the cohort approach is useful in improving *forecasts*. Facts about the past lives of people in cohorts now alive are already established, and these facts can be used to forecast how these people will grow old. Consider the finding (Feinlieb, 1975) that recent cohorts of young people – as contrasted with the cohort to which their parents belonged – showed lower blood pressure, lower serum cholesterol and less cigarette smoking. This finding can be built into models for estimating future rates of heart disease in these more recent cohorts. By applying the theory of cohort differences, forecasts so informed by facts from cohort comparisons can be used in estimating the health and other characteristics of people who will be growing old in 2010, for example, as these people will differ from those who are growing old today.

An important fourth use of the cohort approach is in analysing how cohorts (as aggregate of individuals) fit together to form the changing age structure of the population. Thus in Figure 2.1 a vertical line, as in 1980, is a cross-section slice through all the coexisting cohorts. Each cohort has its special life trajectory of morbidity and mortality. And each has its potentially related unique size, composition, earlier life experiences and historical background. For example, recent increases in deviant behaviour and its health consequences in the US population as a whole are traceable in part to the large 'baby boom' cohorts that now swell the size of the adolescent and young adult strata. Population estimates for the future, as of life expectancy, active life expectancy or prevalence of AIDS, can be refined by piecing together information about the cohorts involved, rather than using straight extrapolations that assume no cohort differences (Manton, 1989; Manton and Singer, 1989). Or sophisticated forecasts of death rates for a given future year, such as 2010, begin with projections using information for each cohort separately, then combine these projections to form the cross-section estimate (Manton, 1989).

These and many other research designs are thus informed by the theory of cohort succession as, for example, in the various seminal treatments by Norman Ryder.

The Social Change Approach

Conceptual understanding of cohorts as fitting together to form the age structure of the population brings us to the fourth approach, to the dynamics of population changes in health. Here, cross-section changes in the health of the population are described or examined in relation to other societal changes. Social change means not only that new cohorts are continually entering the population while others are leaving it, but also that the members of all existing cohorts are simultaneously ageing and thus moving from younger to older strata. For example, it is clear (referring to the series of perpendicular lines in Figure 2.1) that people in the several age strata in one year are no longer the same people as in a previous year: they have been replaced by new cohorts with differing life-course patterns of health with their associated antecedents and consequences. Thus cohort succession is the vehicle producing population changes, including changes in health and disease. Theories of ageing and the succession of cohorts are essential, then, for understanding epidemiological change, and for examining the set of cohort characteristics – such as size, composition or historical experience – that may exert influence on changes in health in the population as a whole.

Changing Size and Composition

The most familiar examples of changing age composition relate to cohort *size*, with the excessively large 'baby boom' cohorts in the United States swelling the stratum of people 65 and over to some 17 per cent of the total population in the year 2000, and thereby increasing prevalence rates of chronic disease. Over time, also, there are numerous changes in the *composition* of age strata, as historical events and population processes affect the health experience of people in the incoming cohorts. For example, as women's longevity has (until now) been increasing faster than men's in the United States, the excess of women over men in the older strata, and the numbers who are widows living alone, have affected the prevalence of osteoporosis, falls and other afflictions to which women are especially vulnerable.

As a striking instance of compositional change within the older strata, consider the proportions of older American men (65+) who are veterans (from World War II and the wars in Korea and

Vietnam) with their war-related vulnerabilities. In the cohorts reaching old age by 1980, only 27 per cent were veterans. But by the year 2000, as more recent cohorts enter old age, the proportion is expected to rise to no less than 63 per cent! Still further into the twenty-first century, the proportion will predictably drop again because members of these cohorts will have died, to be replaced by still more recent cohorts (hopefully) without war experience (US Senate, 1988).

This example suggests, however, how the social change approach – so essential for understanding population changes in health – can lend itself to erroneous interpretation. Just suppose an unthinking researcher, in forecasting proportions of elderly veterans, were simply to extrapolate the year 2000 percentage into the future! Absurd as this seems, many forms of such a 'compositional fallacy' occur, in which interpretations *overlook the numbers or kinds of people* in the cohorts composing particular age strata at particular times. A significant instance of this fallacy concerns changes in the stratum of people 65 and over, where a central question is whether or not, as longevity increases, the health of older people is improving. A frequent answer is that it is not. Yet, this pessimistic answer cannot be simply assumed without regard to the concomitant changes in age composition of that stratum, as the numbers of the 'oldest old' (aged 85 and over) have been increasingly outweighing the 'young old'.

Further Fallacies

Such analyses of how the health composition of populations is constructed and altered bring us back also to the 'life-course fallacy'.[5] The conceptual framework makes clear why it is that cross-section data, which compare an older stratum with a younger one along one of the vertical lines (Figure 2.1), cannot refer directly to the process of ageing. For it is now apparent that the people in these two strata differ not only in age, but also in the cohorts to which they belong – giving very different possible explanatory theories of their differences. For example, suppose it were found in 1980 that people aged 50 are more likely to engage in some forms of disease prevention than are people age 20. Is the difference due to increased awareness of risks as people grow older (ageing)? Or to differences in experiences of cohorts born earlier versus more recently (cohort differences)? Or to mass media persuasion in the year 1980 that is targeted more on the 50s than the 20s (a period effect)? Plausibly, any one – or some combination – of these explanations may be operative. And the theoretical framework shows that there is nothing intrinsic in the cross-section finding alone that can substantiate one of the possible explanations without consideration of the others. To choose among them requires either additional information or special theory or assumptions. So much, then, for the atheoretical doctrine of inevitable deterioration in health because of ageing.

In such ways, theory alerts us to potential misinterpretations and fallacies, and – in the interplay between theory and research – prevents wrong interpretations from creeping back into the theory to confound it.

This dilemma involved in avoiding the life-course fallacy relates to the more general – and perennially confusing – 'identification problem', in which the measured variables are too few to index the number of concepts of substantive concern. In many data sets, including epidemiological records, only two measures are used, namely age and date. However, most interpretations postulate three different concepts: those involved respectively in ageing, cohort succession and historical period, as implicit in the paradigm for analysis of age (Figure 2.1). Abortive attempts to interpret these three from data indexed only by age and date produce serious errors in identifying which concepts are operative.

To circumvent this identification problem, various procedures have been devised (see Chapter 3 by Wolinsky). However, most require additional information – either knowledge or assumptions that certain of the parameters are zero (or some other known value).

Moreover, the theory itself is, in the different approaches described here, not always applied in the same way. When cohort and period are treated as contextual characteristics of individuals, they are conceived like age as among the multiple influences affecting health. However, in the broader sense, the three concepts are in no way cognate with one another. 'Age' is an index for some information about the life course. 'Period' is a surrogate for information about the social and environmental situation at a given time. And 'cohorts' constitute the very stuff of the changing population. In this broader sense, much of the procedural debate is irrelevant. Thus my own view is that the more appropriate solutions are those which do not rely solely on inadequate indicators of age and date, but instead specify and measure directly for the particular analysis the theoretical variables postulated as relevant respectively to the people in the cohorts under study. (For a discussion of this issue, including an example taken from Richard Campbell, see Riley et al., 1988: 260–1).

Complementary Conceptual Models

In sum, this paradigm for analysis of age, complex as it must be, provides a broad conceptual framework within which many fallacies can be identified and avoided, and many particular studies of health can be effectively designed and interpreted. Its utility lies in elimination of implausible hypotheses, and in defining assumptions to be used in statistical models, as described in Chapter 7 by Cox.[6] Nevertheless, as in the foregoing illustrations, the four conceptual approaches derived directly from the paradigm are generally more useful in contributing to theory than in testing it. These approaches, often leading to research that is largely descriptive or exploratory, are more suited to uncovering clues and insights than to establishing proofs. Thus further approaches involving complementary conceptual models are also essential for following up these clues, specifying broad findings in further detail, designing appropriate statistical models, and testing hypotheses. The paradigm is a theoretical setting within which such complementary conceptual models can be located, and special studies can be designed to meet selected objectives.

Ageing as a Biopsychosocial Process

One important complementary model, relevant especially for extending the life-course and cohort approaches, conceives of individual ageing as a set of interacting biopsychosocial processes. This model, with its obvious relevance for research on health, is schematized in Figure 2.2. The psychological and the social processes (for example, as the ageing individual develops coping skills, or engages in beneficial or harmful relationships) are linked to the changes with ageing in biological processes (neural, sensori-motor, endocrine, immunological etc.). The arrows in the diagram simply remind us that all three processes are interdependent; thus, for example, an intervention in one will affect each of the others, and thereby the ageing processes as a whole.

As one example, several studies show how a sense of personal control (a psychological process) helps ageing individuals to cope with stressful events, and thereby improves their social and physical as well as psychological functioning (see for example Rodin, 1989). Even in nursing homes, giving older people a sense of independence and control enhances physical well-being and the likelihood of survival. Other studies are searching for mechanisms that might explain this finding: for example, examining immunological linkages, or showing how older people who believe in their own competence are more likely than other older people to engage in

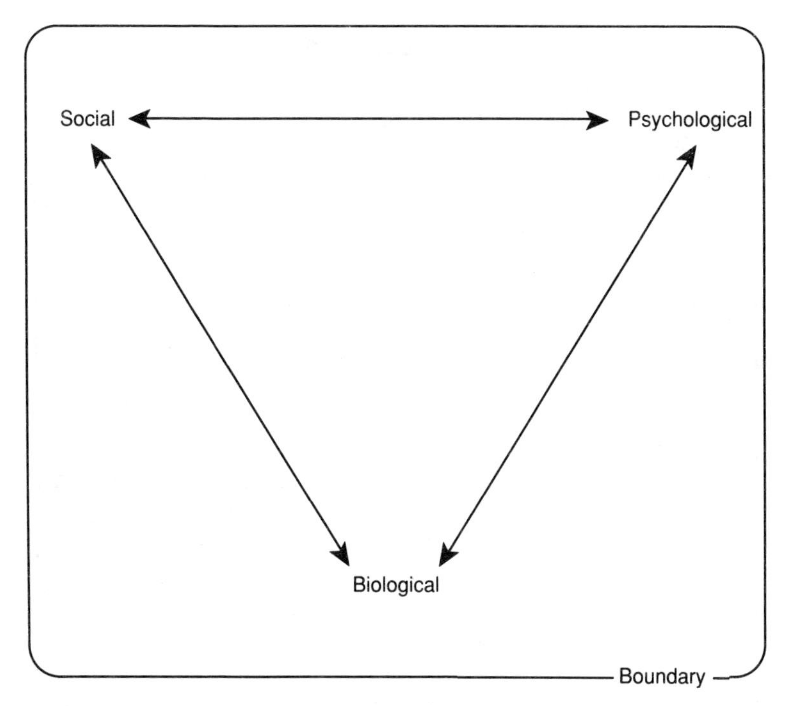

Figure 2.2 *Ageing as a biopsychosocial process*

health-promoting activities. For many research objectives, this biopsychosocial model aids in identifying mechanisms and processes that either prevent or foster particular diseases or disabilities. The potential usefulness of this model, together with procedures for research on the multiple forces affecting health, are discussed in Chapter 1 by Dean.

Age-Related Social Systems

Another important model is especially relevant for pursuing clues from the cross-section or social change approaches. This model takes account of the fact that populations are not mere aggregates of individuals, but consist of *social systems* of interrelated individuals in families, health care systems, work organizations and other social structures (Riley, 1963). The paradigm for analysis of age emphasizes not only people, but also the age structures of roles through which people move as they grow older, and which influence – and are influenced by – successive cohorts of ageing people (cf. Riley et al., 1988). Thus stressful roles in the home or the workplace can affect people's health; and, in turn, increasing numbers of over-

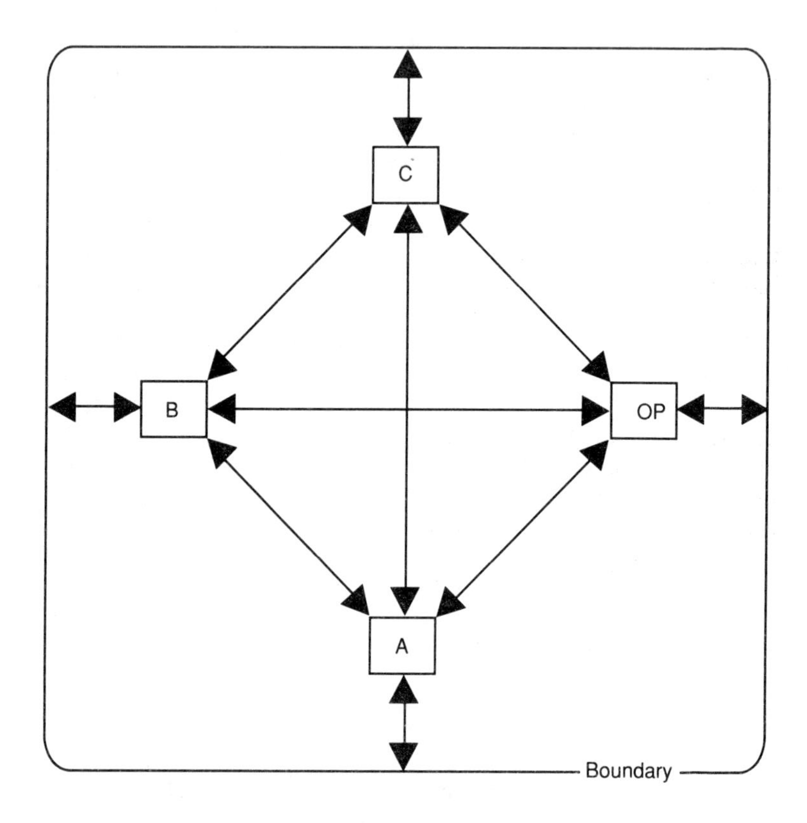

Figure 2.3 *Application of the social system model*

stressed people have serious consequences for the population and the society.

Figure 2.3 suggests a simplified view of the place of a frail or sick older person in the group conceived as a social system – in this instance, a family group. The older person (OP) and three other family members interact with one another, and form a system of members who are interdependent. Within the family system, as one example of the use of this model in research, care givers who are high in expressed emotion (anger, hostility, overinvolvement) are found to perceive the care burden to be greater than do those who are less emotionally expressive. Moreover, the care givers' perceptions of burden have deleterious effects on the patient's functioning; and these, in turn, cycle back to exacerbate the burdens on the care giver.

Applications of the social system model often involve research on limited populations, as in nursing homes or retirement communities. In some instances, however, 'network analyses' are used as complements to national population surveys. For example, a cross-section survey of sexual practices related to the AIDS epidemic can scarcely stop with interviews of individuals: clearly, sexual intercourse involves one – and sometimes several – partners. To understand the multiple factors in the spread of this disease, then, requires utilizing 'snowball sampling' to trace the sexual partners of individuals in the original population sample.

It is this systemic character of both social structures and ageing processes that not only reminds us that cause–effect analyses are sometimes inappropriate, but also alerts us more generally to the dangers of policy or professional interventions that are *unguided* by appropriate conceptual models. The need for models is illustrated by numerous unintended consequences of well-meaning interventions: for example, encouraging everyone to engage in physical exercise, though intended to strengthen joints and muscles, may injure them instead; or tender loving care in nursing homes, though intended as emotional support for older patients, may instead reduce independence and effective functioning.

Summary

This chapter has emphasized the need for broad theory as a guide to research that examines multiple influences on health. A conceptual model (or paradigm) has been set forth that explicates the dynamic force of ageing and the succession of cohorts as integral to the processes affecting health in populations. This model also alerts the researcher to several fallacies to be avoided in tracing health antecedents and consequences, and it implicates complementary conceptual models to provide still fuller understanding. Many of the mathematical and statistical methods for measurement and analysis examined in this book focus – implicitly or explicitly – on particular aspects of the models described in this chapter, or rest on assumptions inherent in them. The hope is that these models will prompt careful scrutiny of all particular research methods and designs as they constitute translations of theory (cf. Riley, 1963: Unit 1).

Notes

1 Works cited are primarily those relevant to the relations between theory and method, rather than to specific substantive findings.

2 Also importantly implicated, and noted later, are the *age structures of roles* which influence, and are influenced by, successive cohorts of ageing people.

3 Personal communication, Robert Garrison, National Heart, Lung, and Blood Institute, National Institutes of Health, USA.

4 In addition to the birth cohorts discussed here (indexed by date of birth), cohorts can be defined by entry into any population (as receipt of a PhD can define entry into the population of scientists). The width of a cohort is defined according to the research objective, e.g. in single years, decades, centuries or – as in the mood swings described in Chapter 4 by Nesselroade and Hershberger – in minutes.

5 Numerous other problems of conceptual interpretation which arise in social research generally occur also in analyses of age. Among them is the 'aggregative' (or 'ecological') fallacy, where collective data for the society (or group, or stratum) are erroneously interpreted to refer to the individual; and also the converse 'atomistic' fallacy of interpreting individual data to refer to the society or population as a whole. (For a fuller discussion see Riley, 1963: Unit 12.)

6 Where age is involved, many of the usual problems of research are exacerbated. For example, in regard to sampling, error may be introduced when frail or sick older people are hard to reach or when young people are away at college. In regard to data gathering, many older people are disposed to answering 'don't know' to standard questions. In regard to analysis, researchers often fail to take into account the effects of migration on the size and composition of the younger strata; or the selective effects of mortality on the older strata (as females, married persons, and those of high socioeconomic status are more likely than their counterparts to survive into old age).

References

Elder, Glenn H. Jr and Rockwell, R.C. (1979) 'Economic depression and postwar opportunity in men's lives: a study of life patterns and mental health', in R.G. Simmons (ed.), in *Research in Community and Mental Health*, vol. 1. Greenwich, CT: JAI Press.

Feinlieb, M. (1975) 'The Framingham Offspring Study', *Preventive Medicine*, 4: 518–52.

Frost, Wade Hampton (1939) 'The age selection of mortality from tuberculosis in successive decades', *American Journal of Hygiene*, section A, 30: 91–6.

Kaplan, George A. and Haan, Mary N. (1989) 'Is there a role for prevention among the elderly? Epidemiological evidence from the Alameda County Study', in Marcia Ory and Kathleen Bond (eds), *Aging and Health Care*. London: Routledge. pp. 27–51.

Manton, Kenneth G. (1989) 'Life-style risk factors', in Matilda White Riley and John W. Riley Jr (eds), *The Quality of Aging: Strategies for Interventions*. Special issue of *The Annals*, 503. Newbury Park, CA: Sage. pp. 72–88.

Manton, Kenneth G. and Singer, Burton (1989) 'Forecasting the impact of the AIDS epidemic on elderly populations', in Matilda White Riley, Marcia G. Ory and Diane Zablotsky (eds), *AIDS in an Aging Society*. New York: Springer. pp. 169–91.

Riley, Matilda White (1963) *Sociological Research*. New York: Harcourt Brace and World.
Riley, Matilda White (1973) 'Aging and cohort succession: interpretations and misinterpretations', *The Public Opinion Quarterly*, 37: 35–49.
Riley, Matilda White (1981) 'Health behavior of older people: toward a new paradigm', in D.L. Parron, F. Solomon and J. Rodin (eds), *Health, Behavior, and Aging*. Washington, DC: National Academy Press. pp. 25–39.
Riley, Matilda White (1983) 'Cancer and the life course', in R. Yancik, P.P. Carbone, W.P. Patterson, K. Steel and W.D. Terry (eds), *Prevention and Treatment of Cancer in the Elderly*. New York: Raven Press. pp. 25–32.
Riley, Matilda White (1987) 'Aging, health, and social change', in M.W. Riley, J.D. Matarazzo and A. Baum (eds), *Perspectives in Behavioral Medicine: the Aging Dimension*. Hillsdale, NJ: Lawrence Erlbaum.
Riley, Matilda White and Foner, Anne (1968) *Aging and Society. Vol. I: An Inventory of Research Findings*. New York: Russell Sage Foundation.
Riley, Matilda White, Foner, Anne and Waring, Joan (1988) 'Sociology of age', in Neil J. Smelser (ed.), *Handbook of Sociology*. Newbury Park, CA: Sage.
Riley, Matilda White, Johnson, Marilyn and Foner, Anne (1972) *Aging and Society. Vol. III: A Sociology of Age Stratification*. New York: Russell Sage Foundation.
Rodin, Judith (1989) 'Sense of control: potentials for intervention', in M.W. Riley and J.W. Riley Jr (eds), *The Quality of Aging: Strategies for Interventions*. Special issue of *The Annals*, 503. Newbury Park, CA: Sage. pp. 29–42.
Shock, Nathan W. (1976) 'System integration', in C.E. Finch and L. Hayflick (eds), *Handbook of the Biology of Aging*. New York: Van Nostrand Reinhold. pp. 639–65.
Susser, Mervyn (1969) 'Aging and the field of public health', in M.W. Riley, J.W. Riley Jr and M.E. Johnson (eds), *Aging and Society. Vol. II: Aging and the Professions*. New York: Russell Sage Foundation. pp. 79–113.
US Senate (1988) *Aging America: Trends and Projections 1987–88*. LR 3377 (188). D 12198. Washington, DC: US Department of Health and Human Services.

3

Age, Period and Cohort Analyses of Health-Related Behaviour

Fredric D. Wolinsky

Introduction

As indicated in Matilda Riley's cogent and eloquent contribution on cohort approaches (Chapter 2), earlier age-related analyses of health and health behaviour were often limited by adherence to the life-course and cohort-centrism fallacies. Indeed, it was not until the mid 1960s that three eminent social scientists serendipitously came upon the same revelation at about the same time. Put simply, they recognized that there was more to age-graded differences than just ageing. Ryder (1965) wrote provocatively about the concept of a cohort, and the importance of the experiential development and sequencing of cohorts. Schaie (1965) wrote insightfully about the relationship between age, time of measurement and date of birth. But it was Riley's systematic and enduring attention to the development of the age-stratification perspective (See Riley, 1972; 1973; 1976; 1981; 1985; 1987; Riley et al., 1968; 1972; 1988) that ultimately provided the coherent and unifying framework. The age-stratification perspective simultaneously identified the tripartite factors of ageing, period and cohort effects, and illustrated how these factors, in combination, produce social change.

The purpose of this chapter is to show how the conceptual logic of the age-stratification perspective is translated into empirical cohort analysis. To accomplish this, the remainder of the chapter is divided into two sections. The first provides a thorough review of standard cohort analytic techniques. The second contains a non-technical review of the more sophisticated and tenuous statistical methods (specifically the 'accounting formula') developed to resolve the identification problem fundamental to all cohort analysis. Throughout the chapter, particular attention is given to the need to focus less on technique and more on theory, if age, period and cohort studies are to be successful.

Standard Cohort Analytic Techniques

The most salient contribution of the age-stratification perspective is its emphasis on simultaneously considering age, period and cohort effects when approaching any substantive issue. The reason for this is well known. To consider any one effect without regard for the other two results in a misleading diagnostic assessment, except in extremely rare 'pure' cases. For example, consider the situation in which the effect of ageing on the percentage of persons who see a dentist at least once during a given calendar year is to be assessed. There is good reason to assume the presence of such an ageing effect. From a developmental standpoint, the progression of dental disease should result in more frequent visits for restorative and replacement purposes. Thus a direct relationship between age and dental contact can be hypothesized, assuming some adjustment for the diminishing returns associated with edentulism (see Conrad, 1982; Evashwick et al., 1982; Beck, 1984; Kiyak, 1984).

Stopping there, however, would be an oversimplification. If it can be assumed that oral health behaviour is a relatively stable lifelong trait secured by early adulthood, then cohort differences reflecting any changes occurring in normative behavioural expectations between successive birth cohorts' formative years can also be expected. Given the dramatic increase in personal oral hygiene during this century, significant cohort succession effects can be hypothesized. They would gradually increase aggregate dental contact rates (see Kiyak, 1987; Wolinsky and Arnold, 1989).

Similarly, period effects on dental contact rates should be expected given the historical introduction of water and toothpaste fluoridation, as well as the increasing reliance on dental hygienists and assistants (Department of Health and Human Services, 1982). The decline in dental caries associated with fluoridation is likely to lead to a reduction in contact rates (see Banting, 1984), whereas the increase in access to dental services brought about by the introduction of auxiliary dental personnel is likely to lead to an increase in utilization (see Wolinsky, 1988). In combination, then, the failure to consider simultaneously period and cohort effects in an assessment of the relationship between ageing and dental contact rates is very likely to yield erroneous results.

The Logic of Cohort Methods

A logical outgrowth of the age-stratification perspective has been the development of a general class of methods that permit the simultaneous assessment of age, period and cohort effects. These methods are generally classified under the rubric 'cohort methods' (see Glenn, 1977; Mason and Fienberg, 1984). They may be further classified into two subtypes: panel studies (sometimes referred to as 'longitudinal' studies), and sequential cross-sectional studies (sometimes referred to as 'synthetic' studies). Both involve tracking two or more birth cohorts over two or more periods. The fundamental difference between them is that panel studies (such as the Framingham Heart Study, or the Longitudinal Retirement History Study) follow the same individuals over time, while sequential cross-sectional studies (such as can be constructed by using the annual cross-sectional surveys of the General Social Survey, or the Health Interview Survey) track different representative samples of the various birth cohorts over time. As a result, intraindividual change can only be assessed in panel studies. Sequential cross-sectional studies are restricted to assessments of interindividual (or more aggregate level) change.

Although the panel types of cohort study have obvious advantages, they are not without their own disadvantages (see Maddox and Campbell, 1985). Principal among these are the opportunity costs of identifying and obtaining baseline data on an appropriate set of birth cohorts, and then continuing to track those same individuals over the next several decades to obtain subsequent waves of follow-up data. Among these opportunity costs are the logistical problems of tracking the cohorts' members, the ambiguities of procuring funding support over such a prolonged period, and the dedication and patience of the investigators to remain committed to such a long-term project. Although recent commitments from the National Institute on Aging to support the establishment of populations for epidemiologic studies of the elderly (see Cornoni-Huntley et al., 1986) are an important step forward in securing such data for eventual public use, limitations in sample size, geographic representation, and the projected number and timing of follow-ups will limit their potential as a panacea.

Because of these opportunity costs, most cohort studies have involved the use of sequential cross-sectional analysis, which is the focus of this chapter. Such analysis is based on the construction of standard cohort tables like the one shown in Table 3.1. The issue under examination in this table is the percentage of Americans who reported a 'great deal' of interest in politics. The table itself consists of data (the percentage so interested) taken from three cross-sectional surveys (in 1952, 1960 and 1968) for each of the seven birth cohorts identified (those aged 21–28 in 1952, those aged 29–36 in 1952, and so on up to those aged 69–76 in 1952). This illustrates an important technical requirement for the construction of standard

Table 3.1 *The percentage of respondents to Gallup public opinion polls who reported a 'great deal' of interest in politics in the United States during 1952, 1960 and 1968 by age group*

	Gallup public opinion survey year		
Age group	1952	1960	1968
21–28	19.0	18.4	18.7
29–36	22.0	22.3	17.4
37–44	24.1	24.8	17.0
45–52	28.6	21.7	20.5
53–60	30.7	28.7	19.0
61–68	33.8	27.8	18.9
69–76	37.3	30.0	23.0
Total	25.7	24.2	18.9

Source: adapted from Glenn, 1977

cohort tables. The intervals between the points in time (that is, the surveys which identify the columns) must correspond in years to the intervals that are used to delineate the birth cohorts (that is, the width of the designated age groups which identify the rows).

When such a standard cohort table has been constructed, the identification of age, period and cohort effects would appear to become rather straightforward. Age effects may be determined by examining *intra*cohort differences (that is, by reading diagonally down and to the right). This allows one to compare, for example, the level of interest in politics reported by a representative sample of the cohort aged 21–28 in 1952 (which was 19.0 per cent) with that reported by a different representative sample of that same cohort eight years later (in 1960) when its members were then aged 29–36 (which was 22.3 per cent), and to compare them both with that reported by a yet different representative sample of that same cohort eight years later (in 1968) when its members were then aged 37–44 (which was 17.0 per cent). This process could then be repeated for the six remaining birth cohorts, with particular attention being given to those ageing effects that were consistently replicated across the different birth cohorts.

Period effects may be determined by comparing the same age group at one time with that at another time (that is, by reading across the rows). This allows one to compare, for example, the level of interest in politics reported by a representative sample of those aged 21–28 in 1952 (which was, again, 19.0 per cent) with that reported by a representative sample of those aged 21–28 in 1960 (which was 18.4 per cent), and to compare them both with that reported by a representative sample of those aged 21–28 in 1968 (which was 18.7 per cent). Here again, greater attention would be given to those period effects that were consistently replicated across all age groups.

Finally, cohort membership effects may be determined by examining *inter*cohort changes (that is, by reading down the columns). This allows a comparison, for example, of the level of interest in politics reported by a representative sample of those aged 21–28 in 1952 (which was, once again, 19.0 per cent) with that reported by representative samples of those aged 29–36, 37–44, 45–52, 53–60, 61–68 and 69–76 in 1952 (which were, respectively, 22.0, 24.1, 28.6, 30.7, 33.8 and 37.3 per cent). Once again, greater attention would be given to those cohort effects that were consistently replicated across all periods.

Although space constraints prevent a detailed elaboration here, an alternative to constructing standard cohort tables warrants brief mention. It involves graphing the relationships. Using the same substantive example shown in Table 3.1, the graphic method would place the percentage of interest in politics on the *Y* axis, and the year of measurement on the *X* axis. The values for each cohort (that is, the diagonal strings obtained in Table 3.1 by reading down and to the right) would then be plotted (using distinguishing symbols), line connected and labelled. If no age, period or cohort effects were occurring, only one flat line would appear in the graph. If only cohort effects were operative, parallel flat lines would be observed. If only ageing effects existed, parallel slopes would be observed. And finally, if only period effects were occurring, a single jagged line would be observed. The interested reader will find an excellent example of the graphic method using cohort sequential (that is, multiple panel) data on the substance use of young adults in O'Malley et al. (1988), and a careful statistical review of the technique itself in Kupper et al. (1985).

The Three Obstacles to Interpretation

As simplistic as it may seem, the interpretation of age, period and cohort effects in standard cohort tables is actually rather difficult. There are three general problems that account for this: sampling error, compositional change and statistical confounding (see Glenn, 1977). It is very important to note here that these problems exist regardless of whether the study design employs a panel or a sequential cross-sectional approach. Indeed, the only difference between the two approaches lies in the methods that are used to resolve the problems.

Sampling error problems in cohort analyses are no different from those faced when using other methodological techniques. Whenever samples of a population are used, the resulting point estimates (such as the percentages shown in the cells of Table 3.1) are subject to sampling error. That is to say that there are implicit confidence intervals around each percentage reported in the table. The magnitude of the confidence intervals depends on the heterogeneity of the target behaviour within each cell (typically measured by the standard deviation), as well as the sample size within each cell. As the heterogeneity declines and/or as the sample size increases, the confidence interval shrinks.

The sampling error problem, therefore, can be minimized when large-scale surveys are available. Moreover, as with other statistical techniques, inferential tests can be applied. Although these are not yet well developed specifically for cohort analysis (Glenn, 1977), the general logic is to ensure that the criteria for statistical significance require the magnitude of any observed effects to exceed that expected simply because a sample was taken. Interpreted conservatively, this would mean that for any two cells under comparison in Table 3.1 to be considered as having different levels of interest in politics, the confidence intervals of the two point estimates (percentages) could not overlap. A more liberal test would require only that each of the two point estimates (percentages) falls outside the 95 per cent confidence interval of the other (see Wolinsky and Arnold, 1988; 1989; Wolinsky et al., 1988).

Compositional change refers to the problem that as cohorts age, they suffer attrition from the death of some of their members. This is especially problematic when cohort techniques are applied to data on elderly adults, in as much as they have higher mortality rates. If the survivors differ from the decedents on any key characteristics under study, then the interpretation of age, period or cohort effects becomes obfuscated in much the same way that experimental mortality plagues the internal validity of randomized trials (see Schaie and Hertzog, 1985). The reason is that as the amount of compositional change increases, it becomes progressively more difficult to partition accurately any observed change between 'true' changes (those related to age, period and cohort effects) and those brought about by mortality-induced attrition.

There are two general means for dealing with the threats to internal validity that are introduced by compositional change. In panel studies it is often possible to analyse the survivors separately from the decedents (see Mossey and Shapiro, 1985; Mossey et al., 1988). Any differences in the parameter estimates between the separate assessments can than be credited to compositional change. Because different representative samples of cohorts are studied in sequential cross-sectional designs, a different approach must be used. Here, various standardization or adjustment procedures can be introduced to compensate for any changes in the distributions of key characteristics of the cohorts over time (see Glenn, 1977). This approach, however, is restricted by the availability of such adjusting or standardizing factors in the data.

Despite the difficulties introduced by the sampling error and compositional change issues, it is the statistical confounding that is most problematic for cohort analysis. The statistical confounding results from the fact that there is a linear dependency in which the basic effects of two of the three facts (age, period or cohort) are involved in each diagonal, row or column comparison (see Glenn, 1977; also note that the statistical confounding issue is frequently referred to as the identification problem, the technical resolution of which (or attempts thereof) will be addressed later in this chapter). For example, age and cohort effects are both represented in column comparisons, because the cohorts to be compared have attained different ages. Similarly, cohort and period effects are both evidenced in row comparisons, because different birth cohorts are being compared at different points in history. And age and period effects are both involved in diagonal comparisons, because the cohorts not only age but age into new historical periods. Thus the separation of age, period and cohort effects by visual inspection of standard cohort tables is difficult unless the observed effects are both pronounced and consistent across all comparisons, which is a rather rare occurrence.

The Visual Inspection of Standard Cohort Tables

Tables 3.2, 3.3 and 3.4 help to illustrate the method of visually inspecting standard cohort tables. All three tables contain *hypothetical* data concerning the percentage of persons in their 40s, 50s, 60s, 70s and 80s who have seen a dentist during 1960, 1970 and 1980. Thus the number of years between surveys matches exactly the width of the age group used to identify the cohorts, satisfying the technical requirement for standard cohort table construction. To simplify matters, each table displays 'pure' (unadulterated) effects related solely to age, period or cohort based on the expectations described above.

An examination of Table 3.2 reveals only ageing effects. As each cohort ages ten years and its teeth naturally deteriorate, the dental contact rate increases 10 per cent. The one exception is that dental contact rates level off when each cohort reaches its eighth decade, reflecting the (arbitrarily chosen) effects of the onset of edentulism. Note that there are no period effects. This is evidenced by the equality of the percentages within the rows. Similarly, the pattern of variation between the age groups within each column is identical

Table 3.2 *A standard cohort table illustrating 'pure' age effects using hypothetical data on the percentage of respondents having seen a dentist during the 12 months preceding the interview*

Age group	Survey year 1960	1970	1980
40–49	50	50	50
50–59	60	60	60
60–69	70	70	70
70–79	80	80	80
80–89	80	80	80
Grand mean	68	68	68

Source: Wolinsky, 1990

across the columns. Thus there are no cohort effects. Indeed, the only effect occurring in this table is an ageing one. That explains why the grand mean remains the same for all three years.

Table 3.3, in contrast, contains only period effects. Here, the increase over time of water and toothpaste fluoridation has resulted in a 10 per cent decline for every ten years. This decline is the same within all row comparisons. It is important to note that in this table there is no variation between the age groups during any particular year. That explains why from year to year the grand mean declines the same amount (10 per cent) as the change for each age group. Thus period effects are analogous to shift parameters in which the distribution by age group within a given year is multiplied by a constant to produce the distribution for a subsequent year.

Pure cohort effects are shown in Table 3.4. Here the pattern is that of cohort succession, in which each new cohort enters the table

Table 3.3 *A standard cohort table illustrating 'pure' period effects using hypothetical data on the percentage of respondents having seen a dentist during the 12 months preceding the interview*

Age group	Survey year 1960	1970	1980
40–49	60	50	40
50–59	60	50	40
60–69	60	50	40
70–79	60	50	40
80–89	60	50	40
Grand mean	60	50	40

Source: Wolinsky, 1990

Table 3.4 *A standard cohort table illustrating 'pure' cohort effects using hypothetical data on the percentage of respondents having seen a dentist during the 12 months preceding the interview*

Age group	Survey year 1960	1970	1980
40–49	60	70	80
50–59	50	60	70
60–69	40	50	60
70–79	30	40	50
80–89	20	30	40
Grand mean	40	50	60

Source: Wolinsky, 1990

with a dental contact rate 10 per cent higher than its predecessor. Note that there are no ageing effects. That is, the dental contact rate of each cohort remains the same regardless of how much it ages. Also note that the changes observed across the rows are in the opposite direction to those observed down the columns. As a result of the cohort effect shown here, the increases in the grand means are identical to those between successive cohorts.

The interpretation of standard cohort tables with 'real' data, however, is seldom so straightforward. There are two major reasons for this. First, it is seldom that a single, 'pure' effect can be found. Indeed, each of the above dental contact rate illustrations is based on theoretically derived expectations for the data. Therefore some amounts of age *and* period *and* cohort effects are anticipated. And that introduces considerable complexity. Secondly, with the exception of the adjustment for edentulism among those in their eighth decade in Table 3.2, all three examples represent only additive effects. That is, the ageing effect was the same for all cohorts and over all periods, the cohort effect was the same for all age groups and over all periods, and the period effect was the same for all age groups and for all cohorts.

But those are not altogether reasonable assumptions. For example, the period (that is, fluoridation) effects are likely to be greater for younger cohorts, because much dental disease is of a progressive and developmental nature. As such, this would be an example of a period–cohort interaction. Similarly, the ageing (that is, deterioration) effects are likely to be smaller for younger cohorts because of their greater exposure to fluoridation during their formative years. As such, this would be an example of an age–period interaction. And the cohort (that is, differential normative expectations) effects are likely to be larger in more recent periods when personal oral hygiene became markedly more fashionable. As such, this would be an example of a cohort–period interaction.

A return to Table 3.1 provides an excellent didactic opportunity to inspect visually what appears at first glance to be a deceivingly simple standard cohort table, even if it does not focus on health and health behaviour. Again, the dependent variable of interest in this table is the percentage of Americans who reported a 'great deal' of interest in politics to Gallup pollsters in 1952, 1960 and 1968. Applying the methods illustrated above reveals two important if not trying things. First, there are no 'pure' effects. Rather, a little bit of everything appears to be happening. Second, what is happening is not occurring consistently across all diagonal, row or column comparisons. This indicates the presence of statistical interaction between age, period and cohort.

There are, nonetheless, several important patterns of effects in Table 3.1. At the most general level, there appears to be a cohort effect, albeit an impure one. Older cohorts who express a greater interest in politics are being replaced by younger cohorts who are less interested in politics. There also appears to be a relatively consistent ageing effect. As a cohort ages, its interest in politics declines somewhat. These effects are joined by an apparent age–period interaction effect reflecting an upward shift in interest in politics during 1960, but only for the two youngest age groups. Similarly, there appears to be an age–period interaction effect reflecting an acceleration of the decline in interest in politics during the late 1960s, but only for those over 60 years of age. Finally, there seems to be an anomaly in that the interest in politics among the youngest age group remains stable across all the periods.

Clearly, this is not as straightforward an interpretation as that given for Tables 3.2 to 3.4. Nonetheless, *ad hoc* explanations (which should have been hypothesized in advance) can be retrospectively fitted to these patterns. The general interest in politics among younger cohorts is likely to be less than that among their older counterparts because of the latter having lived through the Great Depression and the remarkable political and social reforms that emerged from it (see Elder, 1974; 1975; Elder and Liker, 1982). Because the economic and social environments have improved so much and been so relatively stable during the formative years of members of the younger cohorts, they are less motivated to be politically active. The age-related decline in being interested in politics can be argued as consistent with many developmental theories (see Knoke and Hout, 1976). As adults mature, their interests shift from external factors (like politics) to more personal concerns (such as career development and recreational activities).

The three other patterns require more complex explanations, in as much as they represent the interaction of two main effects. An accounting for them, however, can be made. The first age–period interaction probably reflects the special appeal of one of the 1960 presidential candidates, John F. Kennedy, to younger voters. His candidacy may have been sufficiently attractive to the two youngest cohorts to overcompensate effectively for the traditionally anticipated decline in their interest in politics, but only for that one time (see White, 1961). The second age–period interaction probably reflects the extra decline in interest in politics among the elderly brought about by the establishment of Medicare and Medicaid in 1965. Having achieved such important entitlements, the elderly may have turned their attention to other more personal concerns (see Knoke and Hout, 1976). Finally, the apparent anomaly of the stability of the youngest age-group's interest in politics over time may reflect the fact that the first time one becomes eligible to vote is such a novel experience that it results in an unusually keen interest in the political process (see Pomper, 1976).

Regardless of the validity of the above *ad hoc* interpretations, there are two important points to be made from the visual inspection of Table 3.1. First, the cohort analyst relies on theoretical (and not statistical) grounds to explain the general (additive or main) effects of age, period or cohort. The importance of identifying those theoretical grounds prior to the visual inspection of the tables cannot be emphasized nearly enough. Although this reliance on theoretically derived expectations is no different from that involved in any form of analysis (see Knoke and Hout, 1976; Mason et al., 1973; 1976; Mason and Fienberg, 1984), the remarkable complexity of cohort analysis simply makes it all the more important (see Glenn, 1976; 1977; 1989; McRae and Brody, 1989; Schaie and Hertzog, 1985). Thus *the first rule of thumb in cohort analysis is to state explicitly beforehand the theoretical expectations for the main effects.*

The second important point to emerge from the visual inspection of Table 3.1 involves the interaction effects. Although interaction effects may be anticipated prior to the analysis (in which case the theoretically derived expectations for them should be explicitly stated beforehand, just as one does for the main effects), most interaction effects are likely to be discovered serendipitously. Explaining such effects requires a significant reliance on understanding the historical context in which they occur. (Such information can be thought of as a supplement to the data actually presented in the standard cohort table: see Glenn, 1976; 1977; Palmore, 1978; 1986.) Although this is fundamentally no different from the logic used to interpret interaction effects that are estimated in other forms of analysis (such as multiple regression: see Lewis-Beck, 1980), the problem is intensified in cohort analysis because the visual inspection of the tables involves the assessment of *all* possible interaction terms. And that increases the likelihood of identifying false positive (type II) interaction effects in cohort analysis. Thus *the second rule of thumb in cohort analysis is to be very sceptical in accepting the interpretation of an interaction effect, especially if it involves only one or two isolated occurrences.*

Glenn (1977) has gone beyond these two general rules to suggest four more practical guidelines that should govern the confidence expressed in any particular cohort analysis. The conditions under which Glenn believes identified patterns should be given credence include:

> (1) patterns predicted by hypotheses well-grounded in theory, (2) monotonic, or almost monotonic, variation in a row, column, or cohort diagonal, (3) patterns common to several rows, columns, or cohort diagonals, and (4) patterns similar to those shown by other cohort studies with the same or similar dependent variables. (pp. 41–2)

These guidelines serve as a more concrete operationalization of the two rules of thumb presented above. Both emphasize that cohort analysis should be firmly rooted in theory, and that more consistently observed patterns should carry the greatest weight.

Statistical Techniques Directed Towards Resolution of the Identification Problem

As indicated above, the greatest obstacle to the interpretation of standard cohort tables is the statistical confounding or identification problem. In Chapter 2, Riley notes that the heart of the identification problem is the algebraically intolerable situation of trying to solve for three unknowns (the effects of ageing, historical period and cohort succession) with only two known pieces of information (dates of cohort birth and dates of measurement). Although it is generally recognized that the resolution of this issue ultimately rests on the analyst's theory (see Cohn, 1972), much work has been done over the past two decades to develop statistical techniques to assist in such deliberations. In particular, Mason and his colleagues (see Mason et al., 1973; Fienberg and Mason, 1978; Smith et al., 1982; Mason and Fienberg, 1984) have presented what has come to be referred to as the 'accounting formula' (or 'framework' or 'specification'). Despite, or perhaps because of, the considerable controversy surrounding this approach (see Glenn, 1976; 1977; Mason et al., 1976; Knoke and Hout, 1976; Palmore, 1978; Rodgers, 1982a; 1982b; Smith et al., 1982), it warrants further elaboration here.

To grasp intuitively the identification problem, consider the paradigm for the analysis of age presented as Figure 2.1 in Matilda Riley's chapter on cohort approaches (Chapter 2). That figure can be rearranged to illustrate these problems well. Simply imagine that Riley had highlighted, for example, six birth cohorts (or diagonal bars) rather than the three which she labels as A, B and C. Then, assume that the members of these six birth cohorts had been measured on some outcome of interest at each of the first four dates shown in her figure (1890, 1920, 1950 and 1980). By reformatting these data (the cohorts' dates of birth and the dates of measurement) as a cross-classification table and using each birth cohort's age as the cell entries, two important points emerge. First, there would be many empty (or nearly empty) cells. This results from the fact that these birth cohorts only lived through certain periods, and lived through them at certain ages. Thus there would be, for example, no observations either of birth cohort B in 1890 or of birth cohort C in either 1890 or 1920, because the members of these birth cohorts had not yet been born. Similarly, there would be virtually no observations of birth cohort A in 1980, because the members of this birth cohort would have died by then. As a result, it is impossible to say with any certainty how similarly or differently any two of these three birth cohorts would have behaved had they been of the same age at the same time.

It is the second point, however, that lies at the heart of the identification problem. Riley's figure and the cross-classification table that can be derived from it demonstrate that if the year P in which the data were collected (the period) and the year C in which the cohort was born (the cohort) are both known, then the age A of that cohort at that time is unequivocally fixed:

$$A = P - C \tag{3.1}$$

This can be demonstrated by using the example of determining the age of the 1950 birth cohort when measured during 1980:

$$A = 1980 - 1950 = 30 \tag{3.2}$$

Moreover, the same identification problem holds for any of the three effects (age, period or cohort) when the other two are known.

The reader familiar with the use of dummy variables in multiple regression analysis (see Polissar and Diehr, 1982) will see that this is the same kind of problem that occurs there. That is, if the parent variable, say religious preference, has four categories (for example, Protestant, Catholic, Jew and other), then only three dummy variables can be included in the model. The value of the fourth dummy variable, of course, would be unequivocally determined by those of the other three. The three estimated coefficients measure the difference between the religious preference of the groups they represent and that of the group whose dummy variable was omitted (which is traditionally called the reference category).

Schaie (1965) and subsequently Baltes (1968) tried to resolve statistically the identification problem by the application of analysis of variance techniques. Their use of such a two-factor framework (in which the third factor was assumed to have no effect), however, was not plausible. In contrast, the accounting formula of Mason et al. (1973) essentially employs a multiple classification analysis framework that builds on Cohn's (1972) earlier notation. Here, the dependent variable, say dental contact, is predicted by a set of dummy variables representing the age, period and cohort effects. Expressed in the mathematical notation suggested by Maddox and Campbell (1985), this approach takes the following form:

$$Y = k + \sum_{i=1}^{I-1} a_i A_i + \sum_{j=1}^{J-1} p_j P_j + \sum_{k=1}^{K-1} c_k C_k + e \qquad (3.3)$$

where Y is dental contact, k is the intercept, A is the set of dummy variables representing the age categories and the a_i are their regression coefficients, P is the set of dummy variables representing the difference periods and the p_j are their regression coefficients, C is the set of dummy variables representing the birth cohorts and the c_k are their regression coefficients, and e is the error or disturbance term.

Notice that this approach begins by omitting one dummy variable from each of the age, period and cohort parent terms. As indicated above, however, equation (3.3) remains underidentified because of the identity problem inherent in equation (3.1). Thus it cannot be estimated. At this point, Mason et al. (1973) introduce the first of two statistical restrictions involved in their accounting formula. One additional (that is, a fourth) dummy variable must also be omitted. The following is an example of such a restriction in which the additional dummy variable is omitted from the set of variables representing the age categories:

$$Y = k + \sum_{i=1}^{I-2} a_I A_i + \sum_{j=1}^{J-1} p_j P_j + \sum_{k=1}^{K-1} c_k C_k + e \qquad (3.4)$$

Here, it is assumed that two of the age categories will have equivalent behaviour: that is, there will be no difference between them, all other things being equal. The second statistical restriction that must be made in order for equation (3.4) to work is that the effects of age, period and cohort must only be additive: that is, the effects of each must be consistent (though not necessarily linear) throughout the range of the other two.

If both of these statistical restrictions can be made, then the accounting framework will succeed in separating the effects of age, period and cohort. Unfortunately, there is much debate about whether these restrictions are realistic, and about the problems of implementing them. On the first issue, Glenn (1976; 1977; 1989) and Palmore (1978) have convincingly argued that there are many theoretical reasons *not* to assume that age, period and cohort always have only additive effects. Consider, for example, the above discussion of the understandable interaction between age and period shown in Table 3.1. On the second issue, Rodgers (1982a; 1982b) has demonstrated that (a) the commission of even small errors in selecting the 'right' fourth dummy variable to be excluded can substantially alter the obtained regression coefficients, and (b) measurement error can lead to highly inaccurate estimates of the regression coefficients even when the 'precisely correct' fourth dummy variable is excluded.

In the light of such continued criticism, Mason and his colleagues have taken a somewhat softer stance in advocating their approach. This is best reflected by the following statement:

> [The accounting framework's] usefulness appears to depend . . . on strong priors about the patterns in the coefficients as well as specific historical knowledge. Data analysis with unarticulated expectations and meager knowledge may be a recipe for error. A conventional exploratory stance, which works well for models of the additive analysis of variance type, is less suited to the age-period-cohort context, because of the need for identifying restrictions engendered by the inherent interaction among the three accounting categories. (Mason and Smith, 1984: 152)

Fienberg and Mason (1984) have also shown how the introduction of a limited number of interaction terms among age, period and cohort is made possible by employing additional identifying restrictions. These additional restrictions, however, only serve to increase the need to have explicit, theoretically derived expectations for the data prior to commencing the analysis.

Thus there is now general agreement that whether or not the various and necessary statistical restrictions can be reasonably and accurately made, the accounting framework is only a statistical technique (see Hertzog and Schaie, 1982; Schaie and Hertzog, 1985). It is capable of estimating the differences between age groups, periods and cohorts. It cannot, however, explain why such differences exist. That requires a clearly formulated set of theoretically derived expectations for the data. Therefore, despite the considerable attention given to the accounting framework over the past two decades, the fundamental issue of resolving the identification problem remains.

Indeed, after reviewing all of the statistical methods (including the accounting framework) that have been developed for the purpose of separating age, period and cohort (APC) effects, Kupper et. al (1985) are less than sanguine about the utility of such techniques. They conclude that:

> the statistical analysis of APC data is plagued by many unresolved issues and potential sources of error . . . Given these . . . it is our position that such regression methods cannot be said to provide important interpretational advantages over traditional graphical [or standard cohort table] approaches. (pp. 826–7)

Accordingly, it is advisable that any cohort analysis begins with a theoretically derived set of expectations for the data, proceeds with the visual inspection of standard cohort tables (or graphs), and moves on to more sophisticated statistical techniques like the accounting framework only after any patterns revealed from the simpler methods have been clearly appreciated.

Summary

This chapter has shown how the logic of the age-stratification perspective is translated into empirical cohort analysis, especially of the cross-sequential variety. Such analysis simultaneously considers age, period and cohort effects when examining age-graded differences in health-related behaviour. Failure to use such cohort analytic techniques may result in erroneous interpretations of the data, and perpetuate the life-course and cohort-centrism fallacies (see Riley, 1987, and Chapter 2 in this volume for elaboration of these fallacies).

The application of cohort analytic techniques, however, is a reasonably complex process that should not be approached mechanically. Indeed, the use of these techniques requires considerably greater dependence on theoretically derived expectations for the data than most statistical procedures available to the health services researcher. Moreover, even in the presence of a sound theoretical framework, the statistical separation of age, period and cohort effects is not easily resolved. This stems from the difficulties inherent in trying to estimate three unknowns (the effects of age, historical period and cohort succession) from only two data elements (the dates of cohort birth and the dates of measurement). Unless new statistical methodologies are developed to overcome the seemingly intractable identification problem, the analysis of cohort data should always begin with the simplest technologies, such as the construction of standard cohort tables, or graphic representations of the data. Only after the results obtained from them have been fully appreciated should the analysis progress to the more sophisticated regression-based methodologies.

Note

The work reported here was supported in part by grants K04-AG00328, R01-AG06618 and R37-AG09692 to Dr Wolinsky from the National Institute on Aging. This chapter is a much abridged version of the extended discussion of these issues that appears in *Health and Health Behavior among Elderly Americans* (Wolinsky, 1990), published by the Springer Publishing Company. Permission to use these materials has kindly been granted by the Springer Publishing Company, 536 Broadway, New York, New York 10012.

References

Baltes, Paul B. (1968) 'Longitudinal and cross-sectional sequences in the study of age and generation effects', *Human Development*, 11: 145–71.

Banting, Donald W. (1984) 'Dental caries in the elderly', *Gerodontology*, 3: 55–67.

Beck, James (1984) 'The epidemiology of dental diseases in the elderly', *Gerodontology*, 3: 5–15.

Cohn, Richard (1972) 'Mathematical note', in Matilda Riley, Marilyn Johnson and Anne Foner (eds), *Aging and Society. Vol. III: A Sociology of Age Stratification*. New York: Russell Sage Foundation.

Conrad, Douglas A. (1982) 'Dental care demand: age specific estimates for the 65 years and older population', *Health Care Financing Review*, 4: 47–56.

Cornoni-Huntley, Joan C., Ostfeld, Adrian M., Taylor, J.A. and Wallace, Richard B. (1986) *Establishment of Populations for Epidemiological Study of the Elderly: Study Design and Methodology*. Washington, DC: US Government Printing Office.

Department of Health and Human Services (1982) *Third Report to the President and the Congress on the Status of Health Professions Personnel in the United States*. Washington, DC: US Government Printing Office.

Elder, Glenn H. (1974) *Children of the Great Depression*. Chicago: University of Chicago Press.

Elder, Glenn H. (1975) 'Age differentiation and the life course', *Annual Review of Sociology*, 1: 165–90.

Elder, Glenn, H. and Liker, Jeffrey K. (1982) 'Hard times in women's lives: historical influences across 40 years', *American Journal of Sociology*, 88: 241–69.

Evashwick, Connie J., Conrad, Douglas A. and Lee, F. (1982) 'Factors related to utilization of dental services by the elderly', *American Journal of Public Health*, 72: 1129–35.

Fienberg, Steven E. and Mason, William M. (1978) 'Identification and estimation of age-period-cohort models in the analysis of discrete archival data', *Sociological Methodology*, 1980: 1–67.

Fienberg, Steven E. and Mason, William M. (1984) 'Specification and implementation of age, period, and cohort models', in W.H. Mason and S.E. Fienberg (eds), *Cohort Analysis in Social Science Research: Beyond the Identification Problem*. New York: Springer.

Glenn, Norval D. (1976) 'Cohort analysts' futile quest: statistical attempts to separate age, period, and cohort effects', *American Sociological Review*, 41: 900–4.

Glenn, Norval D. (1977) *Cohort Analysis*. Beverly Hills: Sage.

Glenn, Norval D. (1989) 'A flawed approach to solving the identification problem in the estimation of mobility effect models: a comment on Brody and McRae', *Social Forces*, 67: 789–95.

Hertzog, Christopher and Schaie, K. Warner (1982) 'On the analysis of sequential data in life-span developmental research'. Paper presented at the annual meeting of the American Psychological Association.

Kiyak, Asuman (1984) 'Age differences in oral health and beliefs', *Journal of Public Health Dentistry*, 42: 404–12.

Kiyak, Asuman (1987) 'An explanatory model of older persons' use of dental services: implications for health policy', *Medical Care*, 25: 936–51.

Knoke, David and Hout, Michael (1976) 'Social and demographic factors in American political party affiliations, 1952–72', *American Sociological Review*, 39: 700–13.

Kupper, Lawrence W., Janis, Joseph M., Karmous, Azza and Greenberg, Bernard G. (1985) 'Statistical age-period-cohort analysis: a review and critique', *Journal of Chronic Disease*, 38: 811–30.

Lewis-Beck, Michael (1980) *Applied Regression Analysis*. Beverly Hills: Sage.

Maddox, George L. and Campbell, Richard T. (1985) 'Scope, concepts and methods in the study of aging', in Robert H. Binstock and Ethel Shanas (eds), *Handbook of Aging and the Social Sciences*, 2nd edn. New York: Van Nostrand Reinhold.

Mason, Karen O., Mason, William M., Winsborough, H.H. and Poole, W. Kenneth (1973) 'Some methodological issues in cohort analysis of archival data', *American Sociological Review*, 38: 242–58.

Mason, Karen O., Mason, William M., Winsborough, H.H. and Poole, W. Kenneth (1976) 'Reply to Glenn', *American Sociological Review*, 41: 904–5.

Mason, William H. and Fienberg, Stephen E. (eds) (1984) *Cohort Analysis in Social Research: Beyond the Identification Problem*. New York: Springer.

Mason, William H. and Smith, Herbert L. (1984) 'Age, period, cohort analysis and the study of deaths from pulmonary tuberculosis', in W.H. Mason and S.E. Fienberg (eds), *Cohort Analysis in Social Research: Beyond the Identification Problem*. New York: Springer.

McRae, James A. and Brody, Charles J. (1989) 'Reply to Glenn', *Social Forces*, 67: 796–8.

Mossey, Jana M. and Shapiro, Evelyn (1985) 'Physician use by the elderly over an eight-year period', *American Journal of Public Health*, 75: 1333–4.

Mossey, Jana M., Havens, Betty and Wolinsky, Fredric D. (1988) 'The consistency of formal health care utilization', in Marcia Ory and Kathleen Bond (eds), *Aging and the Use of Formal Care*. New York: Tavistock.

O'Malley, Patrick M., Bachman, Jerald G. and Johnston, Lloyd D. (1988) 'Period, age and cohort effects on substance among young Americans: a decade of change, 1976–86', *American Journal of Public Health*, 78: 1315–21.

Palmore, Erdmann (1978) 'When can age, period and cohort be separated?', *Social Forces*, 57: 285–95.

Palmore, Erdmann (1986) 'Trends in the health of the aged', *The Gerontologist*, 26: 298–302.

Polissar, Lawrence and Diehr, Paula K. (1982) 'Regression analysis in health services research: the use of dummy variables', *Medical Care*, 20: 959–74.

Pomper, Fred (1976) *The Voters' Choice*. New York: Dodd, Mead.

Riley, Matilda W. (1972) 'The succession of cohorts', in Matilda Riley, Marilyn Johnson and Anne Foner (eds), *Aging and Society. Vol. III: A Sociology of Age Stratification*. New York: Russell Sage Foundation.

Riley, Matilda W. (1973) 'Aging and cohort succession: interpretations and misinterpretations', *Public Opinion Quarterly*, 37: 35–49.

Riley, Matilda W. (1976) 'Age strata in social systems', in Robert Binstock and Ethel Shanas (eds), *Handbook of Aging and the Social Sciences*. New York: Van Nostrand Reinhold.

Riley, Matilda W. (1981) 'Health behavior of older people: toward a new paradigm', in Delores Parron, Frederic Solomon and Judith Rodin (eds), *Health, Behavior and Aging*. Washington DC: National Academy Press.

Riley, Matilda W. (1985) 'Age strata in social systems', in Robert Binstock and Ethel Shanas (eds), *Handbook of Aging and the Social Sciences*, 2nd edn. New York: Van Nostrand Reinhold.

Riley, Matilda W. (1987) 'On the significance of age in sociology', *American Sociological Review*, 52: 1–14.

Riley, Matilda W., Foner, Anne and Waring, Joan (1988) 'Sociology of age', in Neil J. Smelser (ed.), *Handbook of Sociology*. Newbury Park, CA: Sage.

Riley, Matilda W., Foner, Anne, Moore, Mary E., Hess, Beth B. and Roth, Barbara K. (1968) *Aging and Society. Vol I: An Inventory of Research Findings*. New York: Russell Sage Foundation.

Riley, Matilda W., Johnson, Marilyn and Foner, Anne (eds) (1972) *Aging and Society. Vol III: A Sociology of Age Stratification*. New York: Russell Sage Foundation.

Rodgers, Willard L. (1982a) 'Estimable functions of age, period and cohort effects', *American Sociological Review*, 47: 774–87.

Rodgers, Willard L. (1982b) 'Reply to Mason, Smith and Fienberg', *American Sociological Review*, 47: 793–6.

Ryder, Norman B. (1965) 'The cohort as a concept in the study of social change', *American Sociological Review*, 30: 843–61.

Schaie, K. Warner (1965) 'A general model for the study of developmental problems', *Psychological Bulletin*, 64: 92–107.

Schaie, K. Warner and Hertzog, Christopher (1985) 'Measurement in the psychology of adulthood and aging', in James Birren and Warner Schaie (eds), *Handbook of the Psychology of Aging*, 2nd edn. New York: Van Nostrand Reinhold.

Smith, Harvey L., Mason, William M. and Fienberg, Stephen E. (1982) 'More chimeras of the age-period-cohort accounting framework: comments on Rodgers', *American Sociological Review*, 47: 787–93.

White, Theodore N. (1961) *The Making of the President, 1960*. New York: Simon and Schuster.

Wolinsky, Fredric D. (1988) *The Sociology of Health: Principles, Practitioners, and Issues*, 2nd edn. Belmont: Wadsworth.

Wolinsky, Fredric D. (1990) *Health and Health Behavior among Elderly Americans: an Age-Stratification Perspective*. New York: Springer.

Wolinsky, Fredric D. and Arnold, Connie L. (1988) 'A different perspective on health and health services utilization', *Annual Review of Gerontology and Geriatrics*, 8: 71–101.

Wolinsky, Fredric D. and Arnold, Connie L. (1989) 'A birth cohort analysis of dental contact among elderly Americans', *American Journal of Public Health*, 79: 47–51.

Wolinsky, Fredric D., Arnold, Connie L. and Nallapti, Indira V. (1988) 'Explaining the declining rate of physician utilization among the oldest-old', *Medical Care*. 26: 544–53.

4

Intraindividual Variability: Methodological Issues for Population Health Research

John R. Nesselroade and Scott L. Hershberger

Introduction

Within the past 100 or so years of psychological measurement, the relative emphasis on stability versus change seems to have shifted noticeably in the direction of the latter. Dominant early emphases on the assessment of, for example, human abilities (memory, verbal, spatial relations) and broad traits of personality (extraversion, adjustment), which are presumed to be quite stable and therefore valuable for predicting other characteristics and behaviours, have had to 'move over' somewhat to make room for concerns about changes. Much of the impetus for studying changes has come from the efforts and interests of developmentalists, learning theorists and clinicians.

Coexistence of stability and change concepts has not been particularly peaceful, especially with regard to psychometric and data analysis issues that are linked to the study of these concepts (see for example Costa and McCrae, 1980; Cronbach and Furby, 1970; Harris, 1963). Just as some have argued for the importance of being able to measure and study change, others have asserted that it is a very difficult if not impossible objective to realize (Cronbach and Furby, 1970). Despite the obstacles, researchers interested in the study of change have forged ahead on a number of fronts both conceptually and methodologically (Collins and Horn, 1991) and we are probably now better off than ever before in terms of having relatively rigorous means by which to represent, measure and analyse changes in measurable attributes of individuals.

Different classes of change concepts are recognized in the literature (for example, see Cattell, 1966b; Fiske and Rice, 1955). Labels such as process, lability, state variability and trait change indicate some of the richness of change concepts available to social and behavioural scientists. One distinction that we have found useful is that between intraindividual variability and intraindividual change (Nesselroade, 1991a; 1991b; Nesselroade and Featherman,

1991). The concerns of this chapter centre largely on the former – intraindividual variability.

In contrast to concerns with intraindividually measured phenomena, stability on a dimension is often approached through the examination of interindividual differences. Certainly, this is often the case in population research on health. Stability will not be ignored in the discussion to follow but it will be considered mainly in the context of change.

Cattell's (1952; 1966a) data box, shown in Figure 4.1, illustrates well the multiple modes of dimensions (persons, variables, occasions) over which data might be selected (drawn) in an empirical study. Featured in Figure 4.1 are the three different rectangular data matrices that one can obtain by holding one mode constant and selecting data with respect to two others. An emphasis on intraindividual variability rather than on interindividual differences necessitates the measurement of an individual or individuals across multiple occasions. By and large, social and behavioural scientists have neglected the occasions dimension in the process of selecting data in favour of the persons and variables dimensions.

An emphasis on intraindividual variability implies a concern with states in addition to traits (Nesselroade and Featherman, 1991). Personality traits are relatively enduring individual differences in behavioural dispositions, while personality states may be considered transitory and changeable (Cattell, 1973; Spielberger et al., 1977). Although it has achieved new prominence in the past 25 years, the distinction between states and traits is not a new one. In 45 BC, Cicero distinguished between traits, such as irascibility, and states, such as anger (Eysenck, 1983).

Although controversy has ensued between those who find the trait–state distinction useful (Cattell, 1973; Cattell and Scheier, 1961; Spielberger et al., 1969; Zuckerman, 1983) and those who do not (Allen and Potkay, 1981; Magnusson, 1980), intraindividual research has revealed that an individual's behaviour at any time is a function both of relatively stable attributes and of attributes whose levels vary, even over relatively short time intervals (Nesselroade, 1991b). The traditional prediction schemes of science have tended to use only the former of the two attributes in forecasting future behaviour (for an exception see Cattell, 1979; 1980). In the prediction context, a disavowal or ignorance of the existence of intraindividual variability for behavioural attributes can lead at best to an impoverished characterization of human behaviour, and at worst to erroneous predictions of future behaviour.

When stable attributes alone (interindividual differences) are used to classify individuals, say, on the likelihood of risk for

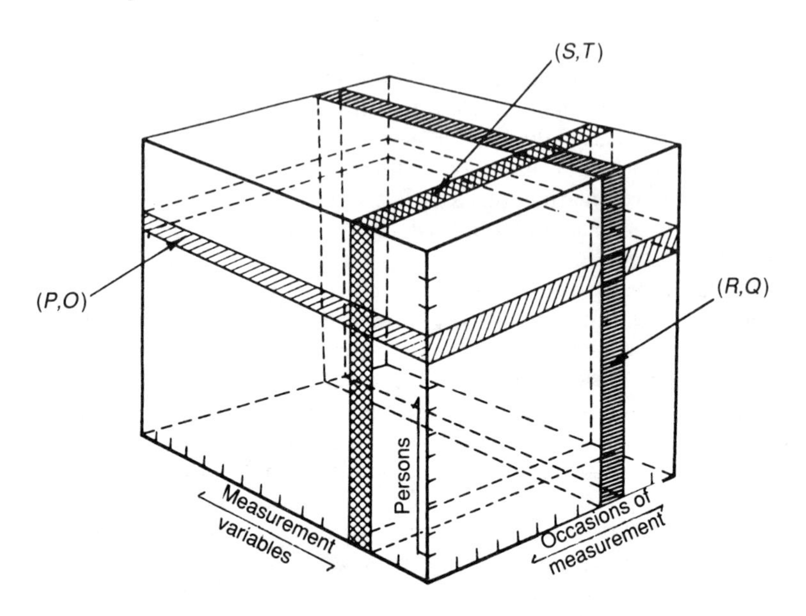

Figure 4.1 *A version of the data box (Cattell, 1952) highlighting data used in various covariation studies. Each 'slice' of data yields a two-dimensional score matrix. The third dimension of the data box is not sampled but is fixed at one element to produce the two-dimensional matrix. For example, cross-sectional group data involve multiple entries from the persons and variables dimensions of the data box, but only one time measurement. This array yields a two-dimensional matrix (persons × variables). Other combinations are discussed by Cattell (1952)*

infection, misclassifications will inevitably arise owing solely to intraindividual variability on attributes (for example, daily nutritional intake) germane to risk for infection but not included within the classification scheme. 'Process' variables which have particular consequence for the individual's ultimate classification on the dependent variable are likely to be overlooked, especially in the absence of substantive theory, owing to the temporal lability often found in the relationship between process and criterion variables. In a similar vein, Dean in Chapter 1 has warned against an atheoretically single-variable approach to prediction in epidemiological research.

We take for granted that interest in change measurement and analysis is legitimate and that available methodologies for studying related concepts, while no doubt improvable, are sufficiently adequate to warrant scrutiny and evaluation. Moreover, we assume that the potential gains in understanding and knowledge base development that might accrue from the study of changes warrant further development of the methods. In this spirit, we will examine some intraindividual change concepts that are believed to be important for understanding a host of questions related to health status, development and other domains of inquiry.

To begin, we will distinguish more explicitly between the two kinds of changes mentioned above – intraindividual variability and intraindividual change. As the labels imply, both will be considered as they are studied intraindividually, but generalization of the concepts to other kinds of unit seems readily possible. Of the two kinds of change, intraindividual variability is less well understood in social and behavioural science and some of its important implications for assessment, diagnosis, etc. are only beginning to be appreciated.

Intraindividual Variability and Intraindividual Change

Elsewhere (Nesselroade, 1991a; 1991b; see also Nesselroade and Featherman, 1991) intraindividual variability and intraindividual change have been distinguished from each other in terms of largely temporally defined features. The distinction is summarized in Table 4.1. There one sees that both phenomena are defined intraindividually but that they are conceptually quite distinct. Moreover, they play potentially very different roles in assessment and classification schemes.

The reader should keep in mind that at any given occasion of measurement, intraindividual variability and intraindividual change can be confounded. So if they are to be separated, one needs to have either repeated measurements at appropriate intervals or measurement instruments that are specific to each of the two kinds of changes. In the writers' experience, this is somewhat unlikely to be the case, but it is a useful notion to discuss from the standpoint of measurement validity.

Conceptual Information Concerning Intraindividual Variability

Although one can find many instances where researchers have essentially regarded intraindividual variability as 'noise' in the system, intraindividual variability has also been the direct focus of concern and conceptual debate. Cattell et al. (1947) helped to formulate the line of research emphasized here with their initial examination of day-to-day variability in the single subject repeatedly measured on a daily basis over many weeks. This line of

Table 4.1 *Distinctions among kinds of variability*

Kind of variability	Change characteristics	Exemplary label	Other key features
Intraindividual variability	Relatively rapid, more or less reversible changes	State, mood	Contributes to characterizing individual at a given time, and thus can confound intraindividual change; can have relatively slowly changing or stable interindividual differences aspects such as rates of change and amplitude of changes
Intraindividual change	Relatively slow changes reflecting processes such as development and learning	Trait change	Contributes to characterizing individual at a given time and across time; central to the interests of developmentalists in respect to both levels or traits and parameters of intraindividual variability distributions

Source: adapted from Nesselroade (1991a) with permission from the American Psychological Association

research, often referred to as *P*-technique factor analysis (Cattell, 1952; 1963; McArdle, 1982; Molenaar, 1985) was instrumental in the articulation of the trait versus state distinction mentioned earlier. The kind of data produced and analysed in such studies are illustrated in Figure 4.1. As shown, the defining characteristics of such data are one individual and multiple occasions of measurement with multiple variables.

Other researchers (such as Fiske and Rice, 1955) also saw the value of trying to formalize the variety of guises in which intraindividual variability had been studied so that it might be more generally incorporated into psychological theorizing. From a living systems perspective (Ford, 1987), for example, intraindividual variability has been examined in terms of steady state variability and its correlates. For the purposes of this chapter, however, we will restrict our attention primarily to *P*-technique data and generalizations of that approach which consider multiple replications simultaneously.

Reviews of both the conceptual and empirical literature offer considerable support for more systematic measurement and study of intraindividual variability as an important attribute of the living, developing organism (Nesselroade, 1991a; 1991b; Nesselroade and Featherman, 1991). An individual's standing on such dimensions, even though it may be different tomorrow, is how he or she is today and, therefore, helps determine his of her self-initiated behaviours and reactions to life events. In this way, such intraindividual variability characteristics are intimately involved in the nature of development, learning and other kinds of less reversible changes.

Empirical Evidence Concerning Intraindividual Variability

A sizeable literature concerning intraindividual variability has developed since the pioneering work by Cattell et al. (1947). Much of our knowledge concerning intraindividual variability has been provided by the application of *P*-technique and differential *R*-technique factor analysis (Cattell, 1963). *P*-technique is concerned with the factor analysis of a single person's score on n variables each measured on N occasions. An N by n score matrix is constructed, intercorrelations are obtained among the n variables, and the intercorrelations are factor analysed to obtain the number of dimensions needed to account for the occasion-to-occasion variability of the individual. Jones and Nesselroade (1990) have provided a recent summary of findings from *P*-technique studies. In differential *R*-technique, N people are measured on n variables on two occasions. The two occasions should be separated enough in time to capture fluctuations. Each individual's score on a variable is a difference score obtained by subtracting the score on occasion 1 from the score on occasion 2.

Programmatic research, principally conducted by Cattell (1973; see also Hundleby et al., 1965), has suggested that for every identifiable personality trait a complementary state exists. This has been true not only for personality attributes presumed to exhibit intraindividual variability (such as anxiety: Nesselroade and Cable, 1974) but also for personality attributes presumed to exhibit primarily interindividual but not intraindividual variability. Human abilities (Horn, 1966) are prominent examples.

If traits tend to have complementary states, then the problem of differentiating them arises in empirical research. Two approaches may be taken to the problem. First, one can try to apportion variance in terms of within-persons variance and between-persons variance. Secondly, one can try to identify key characteristics in terms of their antecedents and label them on that basis (Baltes and Nesselroade, 1973; Cattell, 1973).

The pervasiveness of intraindividual variability on personality attributes calls into question the use of representations that assume a fixed level of the trait. This has implications for measurement, research design and data analysis. For example, the model underlying item response theory assumes that individuals can be located on some fixed point on a continuum of 'ability' underlying the latent trait (Hambleton and Swaminathan, 1985). Individuals are assigned 'ability' scores based on their standing on the continuum. Within recent years, item response methods have been frequently used to analyse questionnaire and personality inventory data. Evidently, one would not want to accept the ability parameter resulting from such an analysis if it does not display constancy across time.

Not only can the level of the trait change across time, but the trait or traits themselves might undergo structural transformation. When measuring a group of individuals across multiple occasions, the occasion of measurement may be considered a selection variable. The term 'selection' in a data collection context refers to the decomposition of a set of data into several subsets based upon one or more selection variables (Nesselroade, 1983). To the extent that selection models hold, there are important implications for further analyses of the subsets of data. For example, if the regression of the common factors on the selection variable (such as time) is not homoscedastic, factorial invariance and, therefore, structural equivalence cannot be assumed (Nesselroade, 1983). Fitting a multiple-group or multiple-occasion longitudinal common factor model with one of the available model fitting programs such a LISREL (Jöreskog and Sörbom, 1986) may be used to evaluate structural equivalence or transformation by testing the invariance of the factor structure.

Importance of Studying Intraindividual Variability

In the light of the substantial number of empirical studies that support the presence of reliably measured, coherent and systematic intraindividual variability, it seems desirable to recognize explicitly its presence in the conduct of various kinds of research, especially research designed to capture important information about the status of individuals on variables pertaining to physical, psychological and social well-being. Although the magnitude of intraindividual variability compared with the magnitude of among-persons variability obviously differs with the attribute under consideration, one should not *a priori* assume that intraindividual variability is of no consequence. The magnitude of the latter tends to be underestimated in relation to among-persons variability because estimates of among-persons variability contain the intraindividual variability to the extent that intraindividual variability changes and fluctuations are asynchronous across individuals. Thus, for example, a possibility that needs to be checked out is the potential role of intraindividual variability in the often reported increase in interindividual variability with age. To the extent that the latter does happen with psychological, behavioural and biomedical variables, one possible explanation for it may be increased intraindividual variability that is asynchronous across individuals. This might signify, for example, the loss of homeostatic functioning with increased age. Nesselroade and Featherman (1991) have recently examined intraindividual variability in the elderly. The preliminary results suggest that the magnitude of intraindividual variability can be at least as large as the interindividual variability for self-reported feelings of depression.

A second reason for systematically investigating intraindividual variability is its potential contribution to the study of stable individual differences. Parameters of intraindividual variability (such as range, amplitude, periodicity, latency and dimensionality) are potentially sources of stable interindividual differences that could be used for prediction as well as diagnosis and classification of individuals. This offers a whole new line of investigatory possibilities that needs to be exploited.

A third reason for conducting research on intraindividual variability involves the differential prediction of the effects of life events. People deal very differently with what are objectively the same events (such as retirement, bereavement or disabling illness). Arguments elaborated elsewhere (Nesselroade, 1991b) suggest that in part these differential outcomes reflect the different status of dimensions of intraindividual variability at the time of the event. This idea needs to be evaluated and, if it is found to be valid, ways to use such information in making predictions, designing interventions etc. need to be developed.

Selected Measurement Issues

Many of the salient concerns with studying intraindividual variability are reflected in measurement issues. The assessment of intraindividual variability, which at current levels of conceptualization involves multiple occasions of measurement by definition, forces consideration of issues about which there is scarcely reason to ask when one attends only to stable attributes and single occasions of measurement. We will identify both some abstract, conceptual ones and some more practical ones.

Distinction between Reliability and Stability

The argument is often advanced that traditional criteria of measurement instrument construction and evaluation need to be examined in the light of one's purposes (see Nunnally, 1967). One specific realization of this general recommendation is to distinguish between reliability as an attribute of the measurement instrument or measurement process and stability as an attribute of the psychological dimension or process being measured (Nesselroade et al., 1986). The relevance of this distinction has become pronounced in part because of the trait–state distinction and the recognition that the time-based characteristics of states and traits can be markedly different. States, in contrast to traits, are not expected to show a high level of test–retest correlation, even over short intervals. Therefore, test–retest correlations, which are often used to estimate reliability, are not appropriate indicators of the measurement reliability of instruments that are properly sensitive to differential changes in individuals. The relevance of this distinction is illustrated with empirical data in Figure 4.2. These data show how sensitive measurement instruments can measure quite labile phenomena in a highly reliable manner. In Figure 4.2, measurement reliabilities for two forms of a state anxiety scale given at four occasions of measurement are all above +0.90, while the between-occasion stability coefficients vary around zero.

It is useful to point out that one of the obvious alternatives to test–retest correlation by which to estimate reliability – the use of internal consistency or homogeneity indices – may be short-sighted. Cattell (1964), who has been one of the more outspoken critics of homogeneity as a basis for measurement instrument construction, has argued that the adequacy of the coverage of a domain suffers if too high a premium is placed on homogeneity. Nor is the answer the use of one-item scales. Nunnally (1967) and others have warned about the unreliability of single items. In sum, the matter of estimating reliability is not a simple one. Cattell (1964) has identified several facets of measurement reliability, none of which can be safely ignored in conducting empirical research.

Validity and Sensitivity to Change

Matters of reliability are clearly pertinent to matters of validity. The notion that one cannot have a valid instrument unless it is a reliable one is not at issue here. Rather, the point is that the way reliability is evaluated must be appropriate to the purpose for which the instrument has been constructed – and similarly for validity.

There is an interesting asymmetry in evaluating measures of intraindividual variability, however. For decades, tests of human

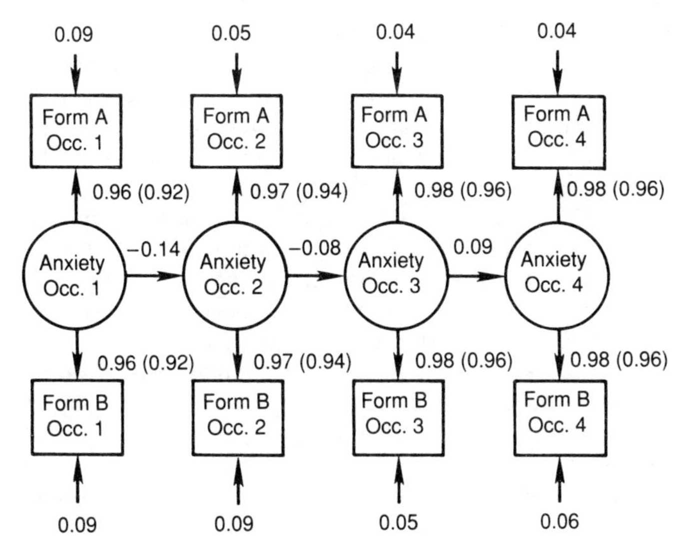

Figure 4.2 *An empirical example of the distinction between reliability and stability (after Nesselroade et al., 1986). Numbers at each occasion of measurement are (from top to bottom): unique variance of form A of test; loading (and estimated reliability) of form A; loading (and estimated reliability) of form B; and unique variance of form B. Numbers between pairs of occasions are estimates of stability of the latent variable, state anxiety*

abilities were said to be unreliable if test–retest correlations, even over substantial time intervals, were not high enough. In measuring dimensions of intraindividual variability, however, if test–retest correlations are high, at least in some circumstances, it is *prima facie* evidence that a measure is not as valid as it should be. The point is that if individuals are manifesting differential changes, even over short periods, then the measurement process should reflect these changes. Thus an aspect of evaluating the validity of measuring instruments designed for dimensions of intraindividual variability is that test–retest correlation behaves accordingly. It is on measures that have this kind of temporally based validity that estimates of intraindividual variability should be based.

Practical Concerns in Frequently Repeated Measures Designs

Protocols involving frequently repeated measurements carry particular risks that are not normally present in, say, cross-sectional measurement schemes. One kind is what was identified by Campbell and Stanley (1966), for example, as reactive measurement threats. The individual may react differently to the measurement protocol the second, third, fourth etc. time it is presented as a function of repetition, thus making it in effect a different test and raising the question of how one can aggregate resulting data to estimate, for example, intraindividual variability parameters; or people may differentially remember their previous responses and this may influence their current ones. Ways to reduce this threat by means of alternative measurement formats have been mentioned in the literature but this does not seem to have been studied systematically. Similarly, there exist analytical procedures whereby one might model such effects and thereby set them aside as a source of variation. Such procedures, however, require an *a priori* notion of the functional form to be modelled or else a remarkable facility for identifying such sources of variance in the context of, say, factor analyses where they might be mixed in with more substantive factors.

Design Issues

Research design issues will be considered in relation to the topic of selection – more specifically, multimodal selection, for reasons that will become clear. The central concern is to orient the reader towards the notion that research design invariably involves choices related to the multiple modes of data classification, such as persons, variables and occasions, and that the decisions made in designing a piece of research carry penalties as well as benefits (Nesselroade, 1983; 1988). The penalties are paid in the coin of limited generalizability, but not just with respect to person samples as is implied in many discussions of these issues.

To orient the reader, another version of the data box (Cattell, 1952; 1966a) is presented in Figure 4.3. This heuristic reminds us that the data we collect in empirical studies are simultaneously classifiable in relation to a number of dimensions. Whose score is it? On which variable? At what occasion was it obtained? When research studies are designed the whole complex of decisions made dictate which subset of data will actually be drawn from the vast data box of Nature.

These design decisions in effect define a series of selection operations that result in one's manifest data. Seen in that light, because the data are obtained by selection operations, the reality of selection effects needs to be recognized.

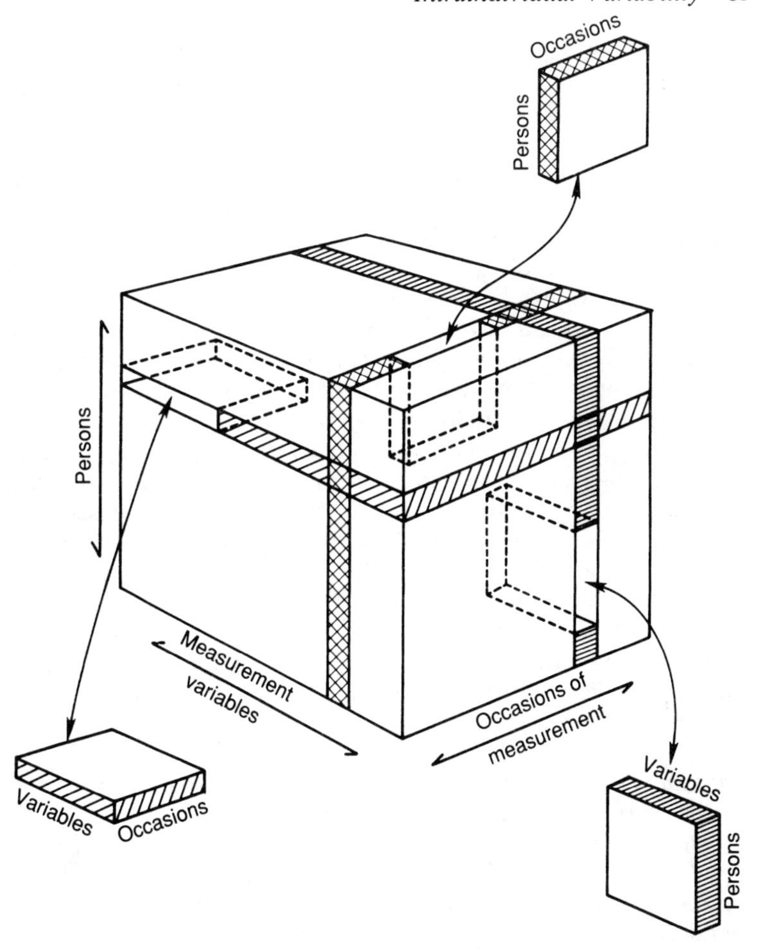

Figure 4.3 *The data box (Cattell, 1952) highlighting the nature of selection involved in conducting empirical studies*

Selection Concerns

Elsewhere (Nesselroade, 1991a; Nesselroade and Jones, 1991) the centrality of selection effects with respect to the study of intra-individual variability has been discussed in some detail. We will summarize those points here.

Selection along the Persons Mode With few exceptions (for example Brunswick, 1956; Cattell, 1952; Humphreys, 1962), the selection of data along the persons mode of the data box has been the most rigorously studied of the various possibilities. Methods and techniques of representative sampling (of persons) have been explicitly worked out and are widely disseminated to researchers. Similarly, the most sophisticated mathematical and statistical representations of selection and selection effects reflect person selection concerns most directly. For example, the effects of attrition due to subject loss in longitudinal studies have been a favourite target of researchers working on selection effects models. Nonetheless, representative sampling of persons from the sampling frame is replete with difficulties, especially so for the epidemiological researcher. As noted by McQueen in Chapter 5, when the representativeness of one's sample is in question, various *post hoc* weighting procedures may be used to correct for deficiencies in the coverage of the sampling frame. Paradoxically, however, the weights so derived are based typically not on the variables which are of primary interest (say, health-related variables), for indeed those are the very variables whose distributional characteristics the study seeks to ascertain, but rather on variables of secondary interest (usually demographic characteristics of the sample). In epidemiological studies, the definition of the sampling frame itself is often in doubt. For example, in both developed and developing countries, accurate census data are often lacking. Because most epidemiological studies will have representative sampling limitations, it is important that work in this vein continues.

Selection along the Variables Mode Selection of data with respect to the variables mode is appreciated by some and seemingly completely misunderstood by others. The advent of structural equation modelling with latent variables in the past couple of decades has helped to focus concern on the choice of indicators or manifest variables to represent latent variables or constructs. It does matter which observed variables are used to represent latent variables of interest. Ill-selected indicators or marker variables do not provide the same estimates of the nature and magnitude of relationships among latent variables as do 'good' indicators, and in that sense the estimates of such relationships reflect the effects of one's selection of indicators.

Attempts to formalize the domain of a concept and notions such as the density of variables through the domain, and attempts to specify how to sample from the domain resprestentatively, have not been well worked out (Humphreys, 1962), although the importance of so doing from a research design point of view is undeniable. Some observed variables must fall closer to the 'centroid' of the concept's domain than others, as illustrated in Figure 4.4 (Nesselroade, 1990; 1991a). It is to be hoped that rigorous ways of

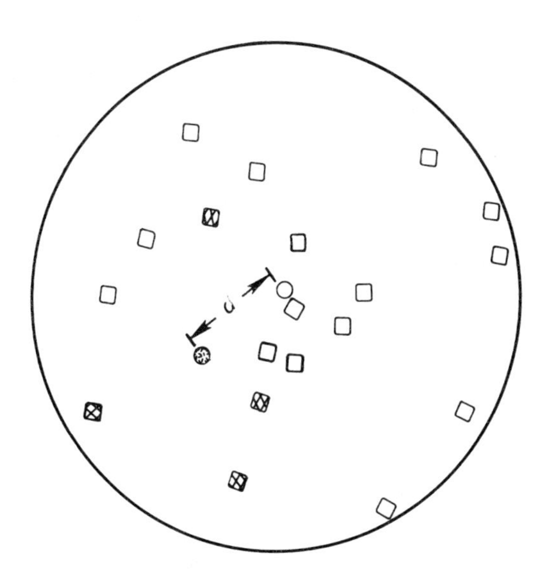

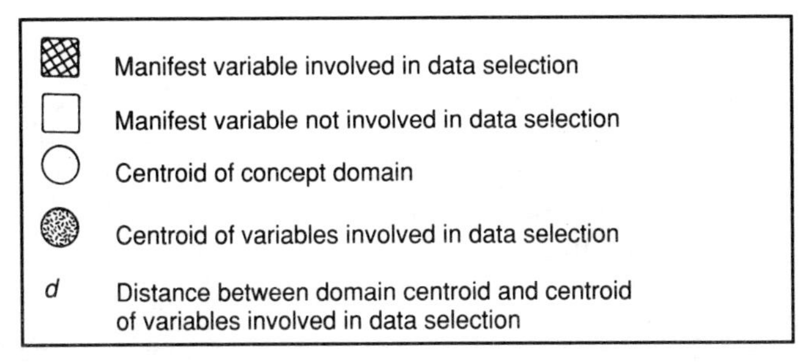

Figure 4.4 *Representation of selection with respect to the variables mode of the data box (after Nesselroade, 1990)*

specifying such notions will become available in the near future so that the design of research can focus directly on minimizing those selection effects that most jeopardize the particular objectives of a given study.

Selection along the Occasions Mode Temporal selection (Nesselroade, 1983) bears most directly on the design of research aimed at the study of time or occasions defined phenomena such as development, change, intraindividual variability and, of course, stability.

Statements about both change and stability involve generalizations across occasions of measurement. Elsewhere, we have found it useful to distinguish between duration and intervals in describing temporal selection and in trying to identify some of the accompanying selection effects (Nesselroade, 1991b). In longitudinal research, for example, interval refers to the time between waves of measurement and duration refers to the number of such intervals or, in other words, the length of the study. Too narrow a selection of duration can result in a loss of important process information, and intervals that are too long or too short will give distorted pictures of the temporal relationships among important variables.

Undoubtedly, serious interpretative consequences can arise in epidemiological research when only one occasion is sampled. For example, when possible causes and possible effects both vary regularly, sampling on a single occasion can lead to false conclusions regarding the nature of causation. The very instability of variables over time necessitates multiple occasions of measurement. McQueen (see Chapter 5) found instability across time in responses to items on an AIDS knowledge and opinion questionnaire. McQueen argues that multi-occasion, longitudinal measurement allows the identification of various sources of measurement error, including wording effects and response biases (such as acquiesence) that might contribute to item instability.

All three of the above examples represent aspects of research design for which decisions must be made. The choices amount to selection on design dimensions and they will inevitably lead to one or more kinds of selection effects that will, in turn, distort the estimates of relationships among variables based on the empirical data arising from that set of design constraints.

Practical Concerns

There is also a set of more practical concerns that need to be faced in the design of research that involves the close examination of intraindividual variability. Some of these were mentioned in the section on measurement. One of the most central has to do with motivation of the individuals to participate and remain in the study. Either differential selection of subjects or differential attrition can woefully restrict the generalizability of one's findings, and the task of repeatedly responding may be an important stimulus for such differential selection. Even in the case of a well-designed sampling plan that epitomizes representativeness, the demands of sustained reporting necessary for estimating intraindividual variability may threaten the eventual representativeness of the data from the standpoint of the persons classification of data.

To illustrate how the different classification dimensions are played off against each other (and thus how selection effects are virtually unavoidable) one might try to minimize the differential loss of persons by decreasing the number of assessments used to estimate intraindividual variability. This is clearly trading off representativeness of the data with respect to the occasions dimension in favour of representativeness of the data with respect to the persons dimension. Or, alternatively, one might decide to use shorter, less demanding measurement instruments but keep the number of occasions at some particular level. Then one is trading off representativeness with respect to the variables dimension in favour of representativeness with respect to the occasions dimension. Or one may keep variables and occasions representativeness high at the cost of decreasing representativeness with respect to the persons dimension, either by deliberately reducing the sample size or by accepting greater amounts of selective attrition.

Statisticians tend to argue most often in favour of persons representativeness, rarely for occasions representativeness, and hardly at all for variables representiveness. Sociologists have been accused (mainly by psychologists) of favouring persons representativeness over variables representativeness, and psychologists have been accused (mainly by sociologists) of favouring variables representativeness over persons representativeness. The point is that these are necessary design decisions and to make them always costs something. To study intraindividual variability with its attendant need for more occasions and possibly more variables necessitates design considerations that are generally in conflict with large-scale epidemiological studies. Thus ultimate design decisions need to rest on carefully evaluated, explicitly stated goals and objectives.

Analysis Issues

Data analysis issues are being covered in this volume by far more competent individuals than ourselves. We would like to mention a few points that are directly pertinent to the topic of studying intraindividual variability. One of the important concerns is the linking of intraindividual information across persons in order to study aspects of lawfulness.

Idiographic Concerns

The study of intraindividual variability emphasizes first what is going on at the individual level. The nature of intraindividual variability may be quite peculiar to the individual in important ways. This may require some data analysis or other manipulations at the level of the person. For instance, patterns of change as manifested in both dimensionality and directionality may be highly unique to the individual. To the extent that is the case, then efforts to aggregate information across individuals will not be very successful until some of the individuality is reduced or otherwise brought under control. Looking for common responses to an anxiety eliciting stimulus (anxiety response patterns) will not be very successful to the extent that there are idiosyncratic aspects to the way individuals respond to that stimulus. If one person tends to respond with increased respiration and another person with increased palm sweating, then aggregating their data will not produce a coherent picture. On the other hand, if the idiosyncrasy is taken into account and both are scored as manifesting increased anxiety, then aggregation produces the kind of consistency that researchers seem to presume, with or without justification, when group data are analysed. Nesselroade and Ford (1985) and Zevon and Tellegen (1982) have discussed these issues at length in evaluations of the role of *P*-technique in nomothetic research approaches.

In addition to calculating elementary descriptive statistics such as means and variances on intraindividual variability measurements, there is a long, if controversial, history of applying the factor analysis model to the determination of patterns of intraindividual variability data (Cattell, 1963; Holtzman, 1963; McArdle, 1982; Molenaar, 1985). As indicated earlier, these studies have provided considerable evidence to support the meaningfulness of such variability patterns. Here, we have tried to suggest the potential merit of trying to incorporate such information in other kinds of empirical studies.

Nomothetic Concerns

The utilization of intraindividual variability information in research employing group designs is a promising avenue for the study of interindividual differences that has not yet been exploited. To do so in large-scale studies will require some efforts to obtain the repeated measures information necessary to compute intraindividual variability scores. In cross-sectional and longitudinal studies this may require designs that permit 'bursts' of measurements on which intraindividual variability scores can be computed. No doubt this will be expensive and will tend to require trade-offs in design parameters as was described above. Nevertheless, if it is decided that such information is valuable, then minimization of the selection effects through broad selections of data with respect to the occasions dimension of the data box can more than offset the selection effects introduced by the design constraints imposed on the data with respect to the other dimensions of the data box.

Summary and Conclusions

Large-scale studies typically invest their resources in representing the persons dimension of the data box as well as possible. Often, these same studies are cross-sectional (one occasion of measurement) in design and involve somewhat superficial measurement procedures (such as self-report on scales consisting of one or two items). The argument we have advanced is that even though research designs will inevitably involve trade-offs in numbers of persons, occasions and measures, it is not necessarily the case that the latter two should be sacrificed in favour of the former. Rather, clearly stated objectives should dictate the resolution of these design parameters. In this regard, aspects of intraindividual variability may be sufficiently attractive to the investigator that the research design will have to allow for more occasions of measurement if such information is to be obtained. Constraints on resources may then dictate that fewer respondents be involved. So be it. The quality of one's generalizations along the occasions dimension of the data box that are based on only one occasion is not improved by increases in the number of respondents; it is improved by a better representation of the occasions dimension. The same applies to the other dimensions of the data box.

Arguments have been presented concerning the need to recognize that there are potentially important data that are not obtained within the usual measurement and design frameworks employed by social and behavioural scientists. We have focused specifically on the assessment of intraindividual variability both as something that helps define the status of the individual at a given time and also as something that distinguishes one person from another across sizeable intervals of time. The first is illustrated, for example, by Jones being more anxious today than he was yesterday, and the second by Jones always being more anxious than Smith. These concepts have not been well exploited yet in empirical research. To do so will require more liberal and perhaps imaginative use of the occasions dimension of the data box. A major point of this chapter is that the time has come to design such measurement concerns into the conduct of large empirical research projects. Looked at from a selection and selection effects point of view, the costs of assuming stability of target attributes and measuring on only one occasion may be every bit as great as the costs of using convenience samples of individuals and the haphazard measurement procedures that abound in contemporary social and behavioural research.

Note

John R. Nesselroade gratefully acknowledges the support of the Max Planck Institute for Human Development and Education, Berlin, and the MacArthur Foundation's Research Network on Successful Aging.

References

Allen, B.P. and Potkay, C.R. (1981) 'On the arbitrary distinction between states and traits', *Journal of Personality and Social Psychology*, 41: 916–28.

Baltes, P.B. and Nesselroade, J.R. (1973) 'The developmental analysis of individual differences on multiple measures', in J.R. Nesselroade and H.W. Reese (eds), *Life-Span Developmental Psychology: Methodological Issues*. New York: Academic Press.

Brunswick, E. (1956) *Perception and the Representative Design of Experiments*. Berkeley: University of California Press.

Campbell, D.T. and Stanley, J.C. (1966) *Experimental and Quasi-Experimental Designs for Research*. Chicago: Rand McNally.

Cattell, R.B. (1952) 'The three basic factor analytic research designs – their interrelationships and derivatives', *Psychological Bulletin*, 49: 499–520.

Cattell, R.B. (1963) 'The structuring of change by *P*- and incremental-*R* techniques', in C.W. Harris (ed.), *Problems in Measuring Change*. Madison, WI: University of Wisconsin Press.

Cattell, R.B. (1964) 'Validity and reliability: a proposed more basic set of concepts', *Journal of Educational Psychology*. 55: 1–22.

Cattell, R.B. (1966a) 'The data box: its ordering of total resources in terms of possible relational systems', in R.B. Cattell (ed.), *Handbook of Multivariate Experimental Psychology*. Chicago: Rand McNally.

Cattell, R.B. (1966b) 'Patterns of change: measurement in relation to state dimension, trait change, lability, and process concepts', in R.B. Cattell (ed.), *Handbook of Multivariate Experimental Psychology*. Chicago: Rand McNally.

Cattell, R.B. (1973) *Personality and Mood by Questionnaire*. San Francisco: Jossey-Bass.

Cattell, R.B. (1979) *Personality and Learning Theory*, vol. 1. New York: Springer.

Cattell, R.B. (1980) *Personality and Learning Theory*, vol. 2. New York: Springer.

Cattell, R.B., Cattell, A.K.S. and Rhymer, R.M. (1947) '*P*-technique demonstrated in detemining psycho-physical source traits in a normal individual', *Psychometrika*, 12: 267–88.

Cattell, R.B. and Scheier, I.H. (1961) *The Meaning and Measurement of Neuroticism and Anxiety*. New York: Ronald Press.

Collins, L. and Horn, J.L. (eds) (1991) *Best Methods for Measuring Change*. Washington, DC: American Psychological Association.

Costa, P.T. Jr and McCrae, R.R. (1980) 'Still stable after all these years: personality as a key to some issues in adulthood and old age', in P.B. Baltes and O.G. Brim Jr (eds), *Life-Span Development and Behavior*, vol. 3. New York: Academic Press. pp. 66–102.

Cronbach, L.J. and Furby, L. (1970) 'How should we measure "change" – or should we?', *Psychological Bulletin*, 74: 68–80.
Eysenck, H.J. (1983) 'Cicero and the state–trait theory of anxiety: another case of delayed recognition', *American Psychologist*, 38: 114.
Fiske, D.W. and Rice, L. (1955) 'Intra-individual response variability', *Psychological Bulletin*, 52: 217–50.
Ford, D.H. (1987) *Humans as Self-Constructing Living Systems: a Developmental Perspective on Behavior and Personality*. Hillsdale, NJ: Lawrence Erlbaum.
Hambleton, R.K. and Swaminathan, H. (1985) *Item Response Theory: Principles and Applications*. Boston: Kluwer, Nijhoff.
Harris, C.W. (ed.) (1963) *Problems in Measuring Change*. Madison, WI: University of Wisconsin Press.
Holtzman, W.H. (1963) 'Statistical models for the study of change in the single case', in C.W. Harris (ed.), *Problems in Measuring Change*. Madison, WI: University of Wisconsin Press.
Horn, J.L. (1966) *Short Period Fluctuations in Intelligence*, final report NSG-518. University of Denver.
Humphreys, L.G. (1962) 'The organization of human abilities', *American Psychologist*, 17: 475–83.
Hundleby, J.D., Pawlik, K. and Cattell, R.B. (1965) *Personality Factors in Objective Test Devices*. San Diego: Knapp.
Jones, C.J. and Nesselroade, J.R. (1990) 'Multivariate, replicated, single-subject designs and *P*-technique factor analysis: a selective review of intraindividual change studies', *Experimental Aging Research*, 16: 171–83.
Joreskog, K.G. and Sörbom, D. (1986) *LISREL VI User's Manual*. Mooresville, IN: Scientific Software.
Magnusson, D. (1980) 'Trait–state anxiety: a note on conceptual and empirical relationships', *Personality and Individual Differences*, 1: 215–17.
McArdle, J.J. (1982) *Structural Equation Modelling of an Individual System*. Report to the National Institute on Alcohol Abuse and Alocholism. NIAAA AA-05743.
Molenaar, P.C.M. (1985) 'A dynamic factor model for the analysis of multivariate time series', *Psychometrika*, 50: 181–202.
Nesselroade, J.R. (1983) 'Temporal selection and factorial invariance in the study of change and development', in P.B. Baltes and O.G. Brim Jr (eds), *Life Span Development and Behavior*, vol. 5. New York: Academic Press. pp. 60–87.
Nesselroade, J.R. (1988) 'Sampling and generalizability: adult development and aging research issues examined within the general methodological framework of selection', in K.W. Schaie, R.T. Campbell, W. Meredith and S.C. Rawlings (eds), *Methodological Issues in Aging Research*. New York: Springer. pp. 13–42.
Nesselroade, J.R. (1990) 'Adult personality development: issues in assessing constancy and change', in A.I. Rabin, R.A. Zucker, R.A. Emmons and S. Frank (eds), *Studying Persons and Lives*. New York: Springer.
Nesselroade, J.R. (1991a) 'Interindividual differences in intraindividual changes', in J.L. Horn and L. Collins (eds), *Best Methods for Measuring Change*. Washington, DC: American Psychological Association.
Nesselroade, J.R. (1991b) 'The warp and the woof of the developmental fabric', in R. Downs, L. Liben and D.S. Palermo (eds), *Visions of Development, the Environment and Aesthetics: the Legacy of Joachim F. Wohlwill*. Hillsdale, NJ: Lawrence Erlbaum.
Nesselroade, J.R. and Cable, D.G. (1974) ' "Sometimes it's okay to factor

difference scores" – the separation of trait and state anxiety', *Multivariate Behavioral Research*, 9: 273–82.

Nesselroade, J.R. and Featherman, D.L. (1991) 'Intraindividual variability in older adults' depression scores: some implications for developmental theory and longitudinal research', in D. Magnusson, L. Bergman, G. Rudinger and B. Torestad (eds), *Stability and Change: Methods and Models for Data Treatment*. London: Cambridge University Press.

Nesselroade, J.R. and Ford, D.H. (1985) '*P*-technique comes of age: multivariate, replicated, single-subject designs for research on older adults', *Research on Aging*, 7: 46–80.

Nesselroade, J.R. and Jones, C.J. (1991) 'Multi-model selection effects in the study of adult development: a perspective on multivariate, replicated, single-subject repeated measures', *Experimental Aging Research*, 17: 21–7.

Nesselroade, J.R., Pruchno, R. and Jacobs, A. (1986) 'Reliability and stability in the measurement of psychological states: an illustration with anxiety measures', *Psychologische Beitraege*, 28: 255–64.

Nunnally, J.C. (1967) *Psychometric Theory*. New York: McGraw-Hill.

Spielberger, C.D., Gorsuch, R.L. and Lushene, R. (1969) *The State–Trait Anxiety Inventory (STAI) Test Manual, Form X*. Palo Alto, CA: Consulting Psychologists Press.

Spielberger, C.D., Lushene, R.E and McAdoo, W.G. (1977) 'Theory and measurement of anxiety states', in R.B. Cattell and R.M. Dreger (eds), *Handbook of Modern Personality Theory*. New York: Wiley.

Zevon, M.A. and Tellegen, A. (1982) 'The structure of mood change: an idiographic/nomothetic analysis', *Journal of Personality and Social Psychology*, 43: 111–22.

Zuckerman, M. (1983) 'The distinction between trait and state scales is not arbitrary: comment on Allen and Potkay's "On the Arbitrary distinction between traits and states" ', *Journal of Personality and Social Psychology*, 44: 1083–6.

5

A Methodological Approach for Assessing the Stability of Variables Used in Population Research on Health

David V. McQueen

Introduction

One of the established approaches to understanding complex population phenomena has been to carry out survey research. Although the survey approach may appear fairly established and straightforward, it remains a rather complicated endeavour. There are numerous well-understood techniques for design, data collection and analysis, but many of these have changed little over the years. Thus the most frequently used design is still a cross-section survey with some approximation to a random sampling process; the common method of data collection is by personal interview; and the general analysis is by correlation and cross-tabulations. This is the prevalent form of survey research in health studies. It is seen in countless local, regional and national surveys on lifestyle, risk factor and needs assessment. This approach is accompanied by a number of underlying assumptions, notably the implicit notion of an experimental design. Thus one sees the emphasis on so-called baseline surveys and/or a series of such surveys. Because this approach accepts the underlying canons of probabilistic thinking it has within it may assumptions such as: (1) a well-circumscribed, known (or potentially knowable) population; (2) variables to be measured which have an approximately known value; (3) control over the data collection process, as for example by a consistent interviewing procedure; and (4) techniques to reduce, eliminate or explain survey error. The numerous technical and practical problems which underly each of these assumptions have been elaborated in critical methodological literature of recent years (Lieberson, 1984). Unfortunately this critique is found largely within the rather esoteric realm of the sociological methodologists; their often mathematically sophisticated arguments rarely reach the many health science practitioners carrying out survey research routinely in the field. Therefore it is hardly surprising that the more severe criticisms of widely used methods and attempts to further develop other methods are seldom applied by the practitioner, and the standard series of cross-sectional designs remains the dominant approach in survey research on health.

This apparent failure of critical methodological discussions to reach many health researchers is all the more unfortunate because of the changing theoretical underpinning of health services research. In recent years the emphasis in social science research has moved to the consideration of variables of process. Many of the variables and ideas of concern to sociomedical researchers are dynamic rather than static. Variables such as coping, social support and empowerment are concerned with dynamic processes. In turn these dynamic processes take place over time. Unfortunately the mathematical and statistical techniques of social scientists such as Blalock (1969), Coleman (1964; 1990) and Tuma and Hannan (1984), which could provide innovative dynamic perspectives to data collection and analysis, remain relatively unused or unseen by many health researchers. In addition, the science skills, statistical and mathematical, behind these techniques are outside the training of most health researchers. This may be because they stem largely from a mathematical base. The graphical analyses and techniques addressed elsewhere in this book are simply examples of the kind of new approaches which can be brought to bear on the analysis of survey data.

The move from static to dynamic concepts has further implications which are perhaps less appreciated. While analytical capacities have improved over the years, research designs have remained largely static, including the methods of sampling, data collection and assessment of error. Thus although the technology of recent years has had considerable impact on options for the analysis of survey data, it has had relatively less impact on how data are collected. Part of the reason has been the inability of survey research, with its cumbersome data collection procedures, to collect data rapidly and in temporal relation to actual processes occurring in the population and among individuals. That is, the standard data collection approaches lack a dynamic measure of the element of time.

A major implication of collecting data continuously is that the dynamics of the variables measured can be more fully appreciated and evaluated. For example, traditionally many health surveys have been limited to estimating the prevalence of an attitude or behaviour at one time. This tells one little about the dynamics of the attitude on behaviour in the population. Even further analysis which considers this estimate in relation to other characteristics of the population such as age, race and socioeconomic status yields little insight into the dynamics of those attitudes or behaviours in the subanalysed population groups. Adding a longitudinal design based on a series of cross-sectional surveys gives more insight into the dynamics of the measured attitudes and behaviours. For example, one can discuss *trends* in prevalence and apparent absolute change from one time to another. Nevertheless, the full dynamics of the measured attitudes and behaviours are not revealed unless a continuous design is employed. In particular what is missing from the full dynamic picture is an understanding of the path of variability over time in the measured variable. In the research described below this translates into a concern with examining the stability (or instability) of attitudinal and behavioural variables as they reveal themselves in survey data collected continuously.

A Continuous Data Stream: Theoretical Aspects

The notion of a continuous stream of data is unusual in relation to health and lifestyle variables because such data collection has not been a tradition in the sociomedical sciences. There are many sciences which collect and/or study data collected continuously, notably economics, physics, biology and geology. In each of these sciences there is the idea that long periods are often necessary before any significant changes in a large system occur. Of course changes are always occurring at micro levels, but quite often the level of interest is at a more macro level. Geological phenomena are classic in this sense: observable changes at the macro level may take hundreds, thousands or even millions of years. One expects changes in the social system to take place much more rapidly, but that is probably due to our observation level which is focused on the individual. When one considers the macro level of social systems, changes are generally more subtle, slower and therefore less perceptible. Consider the notion of a 'sick society' in contrast to a 'sick individual'. In the individual, illness may be subtle, but more often it is perceptible to the individual and in many cases to outside experts such as physicians. Furthermore the dynamics of the disease are readily discernible, and diagnosis and prognosis are developed to a high art. The signs and symptoms of a sick society are more diffuse and more debatable, and often do not occur at a rapid pace. Thus the debate about whether a particular country or society is in decline is always complicated and the case for decline is difficult to prove.

From the standpoint of health-related variables, the solution to some of the technical problems associated with health research which takes a 'dynamic' perspective is very important. If it is argued that behavioural patterns and population variables related to health express themselves in continuously collected data in a dynamic way, fluctuating and changing over time, then the case for a strong conceptual fit between theory and method is very good. But the implications for data collection are that it must be carried out for a considerable time. It also implies that what constitutes a completed section of this long-term process is very much dependent on how the various variables in the study manifest themselves over time (Tanur, 1983).

The use of continuous data collection introduces the recurrent question of the unit of observation. To date most longitudinal data have emphasized the change in individual behaviour over time, concentrating both on real time and on time in an individual lifespan. This, of course, emphasizes the individual at the expense of other units of observation, notably the collectivity. This individualistic approach tends to negate the idea of behaviours as phenomena themselves which change in character and structure over time within populations. Despite the richness of longitudinal data collection, health research has not addressed the collection and analysis of data on non-individual units. One implication of continuous data collection on health-related opinions, attitudes and behaviours is that these may be expressed over time as a collective notion even though the individual may be the source of report at any discrete point in the data collection process. The results of collecting data continuously with the new technology are only beginning to emerge. Nonetheless, many findings emerging from the analysis of continuous data challenge the assumptions of the traditional approaches and, therefore, seriously question the basis for doing research on dynamic questions.

Data Collection and the Move to a Concept of Total Survey Error

Error has always been a concern in survey research, but increasingly researchers have turned to the concept of total survey error (Groves, 1989). Part of the reason for this is that, coterminously with the concern with error, several events have occurred which exacerbate the difficulties of survey research. Some of these problems raise general questions regarding error, as for example the use of computer assisted telephone interviewing (CATI) and the generalized reduction in public cooperation rates with researchers (Steeh, 1981). More importantly for our consideration is the need for data which integrate various levels of variables; the notion that variables sit in a larger context; and the development of new theoretical perspectives, for example dynamic models which challenge many fundamental assumptions of measurement which ultimately impinge on error.[1]

The idea of total survey error combines many different aspects of error. It is concerned with error arising from non-response and coverage, but these are commonly treated error sources. It is also concerned with sampling error, but adds the dimension that it takes into account sampling error over many trials in a survey. This sampling error may vary from trial to trial. For example, in continuously collected data a sampling strategy may be to draw a sample on a monthly basis. Thus one has a series of samples of trials with slightly varying sampling error. Furthermore respondents are expected to vary in their response to questions over time, leading to response variance. A further feature of the concept of total survey error is the accounting for error arising from interviewer variance over the course of a survey or series of trials. In short the idea of total survey error encompasses a broader concept of error than that generally used in single cross-sectional survey designs.

Continuous data collection presents numerous methodological challenges to the concept of total survey error. For reasons of cost, efficiency, interview control and data flow management the telephone has become a major instrument for data collection and is the instrument of choice to collect data continuously. Nonetheless, telephone ownership is limited, and whereas all modes of data collection have their numerous sources of error, these are familiar errors. To many researchers the literature on the reduction of bias in telephone interviewing, or the literature on the validity and reliability of health data collected by telephone, is still relatively unfamiliar ground. This unfamiliarity has decreased in recent years with the shift to the problem of total survey error arising from sampling variability, non-sampling variability, response effects and non-participation effects. The latter is a special problem, as both American and European studies have noted an increase in non-response rates for all types of interviewing. Many techniques such as call-backs, encouragement and promise of confidentiality have been used with varying success; in addition, statistical techniques such as weighting for missing data and imputation techniques have been developed to account for data collection variability.

Table 5.1 illustrates some of the sources of error in a population survey and how they might be treated in continuously collected data. The error sources, shown in the first column, merely represent some of the key areas for error and have been chosen because of their amenability to adjustment. The estimate of amenability is

Table 5.1 *Some sources of error and their amenability to adjustment*

Error source	Method of adjustment	Amenability[1]
Non-response	Mixed statistical and non-statistical	Slight
Coverage	Statistical	Slight
Sampling	Statistical	High
Interviewer	Management, statistical	Moderate
Respondent	Continuous data	Moderate
Instrument	Rewording analysis	Moderate
Costs	Management, statistical	Moderate

[1] Based on continuously collected data.

based on five years' experience with data collected continuously and discussions with other survey researchers; thus the assessment of amenability is a consideration of empirical experience and subjective evaluations. The important thing to note is that the first three sources of error are largely errors related to sampling and treatable by statistical methods, and the second four are chiefly errors related to data collection procedures and treatable through a variety of methods which are not statistical and relate to the data collection process itself. It is probably safe to assert that the first three have been seen as problems for statisticians and the second four as problems for survey researchers with social science backgrounds, chiefly sociologists. Indeed, the arguments put forward by Groves (1989) lead to a distinction among survey researchers between those who wish to reduce error and those who wish to explain error; by and large statisticians think about error in terms of bias, whereas sociologists think about variance. The distinction between bias and variance reduction and explanation is important because it stems from the very fundamental ethos of the disciplines and perhaps underlies some of the difficulties which often arise in communication between statisticians and social scientists.

A further illustration of the different perceptions comes from the notion of reliability. The survey researcher concerned with statistical repeatability hopes to construct an item which will be answered in exactly the same way by the same person time after time, *ceteris paribus*. That is, if a respondent is asked how healthy she feels, and she feels very good on Monday and feels the same way on Friday, then in both cases 'very good' is the appropriate response, and the question item is considered reliable if the same response category is ticked on both days. But in practice, that is when the respondent actually fills out the item, she may tick this highly 'reliable' item differently on the two days. Although this may appear as a challenge to the reliability of the question item, the differential ticking of the item may be due to some small conceptual shift about the meaning of the words 'very good' over the period between the two questions, even though there is little apparent or detectable difference in the person's overall view of how healthy she feels. For the social scientist it is often the discrepancy between two responses which need to be explained. This type of conceptual shift problem which challenges reliability is particularly pertinent for longitudinal data collected on the same individuals over time; it is less of a problem for continuously collected data on aggregate behaviours because these reporting differences probably constitute randomly distributed bias.

It is a similar argument with validity. It has long been asserted by those concerned with psychometric measurement that construct validity is an exceedingly problematic concept (Nunnally, 1978) in measurement. More recent writings on reflexivity and research suggest that constructs tell us mostly about the structure and design of the researchers and the research rather than about any conceptual reality in the real world (Steier, 1991). Nonetheless, the idea persists in survey research that one can write questionnaire items which are highly conceptual and expect the conceptual domains of these items to remain relatively well circumscribed and stable each time they are asked by an interviewer and each time they are answered by a respondent. Furthermore it is postulated that at the point of analysis the research can reach into the data and extract the expected constructs. This is, however, the theoretical expectation of the methodologist.

From an epistemological perspective the issue of construct validity centres on ideas of concept formation. Concept formation remains a distinguished yet highly debated area in the philosophy of science. A distinguishing feature of the debate centres on the meaning of concepts and whether or not that meaning can ever be reduced to something which can be measured. For many the search of what social scientists term 'construct validity' would be elusive; the best one could hope for would be 'operational' measures of concepts. In continuously collected data the researcher is more explicitly controlling the data collection process. Thus the data tend to be more descriptive of events occurring in time reported by individuals. The events collectively, at the aggregate level, are the subject of analysis.

For those social scientists who have been influenced by the growing qualitative research approach, the idea that a conceptual notion can be well circumscribed and remain fundamentally stable is disappearing. Thus signs of minor shifts in conceptual meaning which might be seen as errors in data may in fact only be markers of the level of stability of the concept in the cognition of the individuals participating in the survey.[2] Thus the valid measure of a concept which has instability over time requires a measuring instrument which captures that instability. This requires attention both to the questionnaire design and to the data collection process, for both are part of the measuring instrument.

These issues of error arising around reliability and validity merely illustrate that different sources of error place differing demands on researchers. If one views the survey research effort as a collective one, carried out by a team of people, then dealing with error requires a number of skills and disciplines. The reality is that the data collection process takes on its own dimensions and the research teams are limited in their skills and ability to address and cope with all the potential sources of error in the survey process. That is undoubtedly why the option often taken in survey research is to address those errors which can be corrected statistically via some well-established practice. Nevertheless there are problems which impinge on the success of this accepted practice. These problems arise when a broader idea of error is taken into consideration and a more reflexive perspective is taken. This approach requires a considerable rethinking of the relationship between theory, data and the method of data collection.

Consider the fundamental problem of sampling and representativeness which is usually further exacerbated by the problem of coverage (some persons are not part of the sampling frame). The representativeness problem is often addressed by post-survey weighting procedures and is transformed into a problem of analysis. In standard procedures the sample characteristics are compared with population characteristics as gleaned from a criterion source (for example an official census) and the estimates from the sample are weighted in order to be closer in value to the population parameters. This is a fine procedure, technically interesting, but sociologically dismissive because the weights are based on the variables in the survey which are of relatively secondary interest, usually simple demographic characteristics. The focus of much survey research, particularly that in health, is on variables which have no clearly known criterion distribution in the population. A good example is the number of sexual partners reported by a respondent over a particular period. In this case the researcher must rely entirely on the number stated by the respondent. The number obtained by the data collection process will vary significantly in relation to how the question is asked, the response categories allowed, and the time of recall. This is a fundamental measurement problem which becomes even more complicated when one tries to assess the veracity of the respondent. Given the complexity of estimating the balance between measurement error, accuracy and veracity in the response to this basic question, it is clearly very difficult to determine what is the appropriate weighting factor with respect to this item. Thus the researcher moves very quickly to a problem of error which combines problems of coverage, instrumentation and weighting.

The overemphasis on the post-survey statistical aspect of surveys has been at the expense of treating errors during data collection itself, notably through data collection management considerations. Nonetheless, a significant source of error in surveys comes from the 'social dynamics' of the questionnaire and from problems in the management of the data collection. Some aspects of the total error picture are included in Table 5.1. Ultimately, survey error is affected by the quality and efficiency of the data collection process and the amount of resources available to address issues of error which arise during a study. That is why cost becomes an important consideration in assessment of error (Groves, 1989). Simply put, there is a new budgetary concern if one wishes to consider error issues during the data collection time itself. In the collection of data continuously it is obvious that the timely review of error sources while data are being collected is very important, and is another dimension of this approach which differs from adjusting errors *post hoc* in cross-sectional surveys.

A Further Rationale for Collecting Data Continuously

In order to study behavioural variables measured at the population level which are considered dynamic and in a state of flux or subject to change over time, one needs to collect data which approximates real time events in the population. In practice this means maintaining a data collection system which carries out interviewing on a daily basis. An example is the CATI-based survey system at the Research Unit in Health and Behavioural Change, Edinburgh, where data have been collected daily, excluding holidays and Sundays, since July 1987.[3]

The rationale for such a continuous data collection system arose out of theoretical and methodological concerns. The theoretical reasons have been discussed in detail elsewhere (RUHBC, 1989). They may be summarized briefly as being related to the concern in sociological theory, developed largely in the 1970s and 1980s, with notions that population level behavioural variables measured through individuals operate as part of processes embedded in a larger (macro) social context. Furthermore, the study of behavioural change implies a dynamic theory. The methodological reasons go back to the earlier work of Coleman (1964) on the mathematical analysis of change, and to Tuma and Hannan's (1984) more recent work on social dynamical models and methods.[4]

Given that behavioural variables used in health research are very dynamic, an appropriate data collection method should seek to provide data which describe this dynamism. The data collection procedure is analogous to an instrument which should be tuned until it collects the data in a robust manner, so that variance in the data is not coming from variance in the data collection procedure. Thus the data collection procedure, as an instrument, needs running-in time, that is time to warm up and stabilize. Furthermore, as it runs, its peculiarities as an instrument become familiar to those carrying out the research. Thus the research team is better equipped to distinguish variability in the data which is attributable to the instrument, to the data collection process or to the interviewer.

Continuously Collected Data: Practical Aspects

Thus the argument is that the development of CATI has not only changed the data collection process, but also allowed some innovative approaches to issues related to error and to the analysis of behavioural change. Through the use of daily interviewing with a random digit dialling procedure it is possible to obtain a stream of data which approximates a continuous data set incorporating a day-in, day-out measure of behaviour in the population. There are many critical technical issues to be considered but the main issues revolve around sampling, measurement and data management. Sampling is a challenge because of the time constraints on the sampling frame, that is one can conceptualize the sample as one being taken continuously in time. This is in contrast to samples which are taken solely on the basis of static considerations such as areas or fixed populations. When CATI is used with a random digit dialling technique, drawing the sample and data collection become coterminous and integrated.

Data management becomes a major consideration in the collection of data which are time bound and/or continuous. Day-to-day management becomes a concern for the researcher. For example, in traditional cross-sectional survey research the period of data collection often precedes the conversion of the data for analysis. That is, questionnaires are stockpiled and then coded, and when coding is completed a finished data file is processed. However, in the use of CATI to collect data in very short discrete periods on a regular basis over a long time, the brief periods, even as short as a few hours, which lie between data collection times may be used to review the data received recently in order to verify and tune the data collection procedure. After a longer period the researcher may make strategic adjustments in the actual questions asked. In short the data collection and analysis are very integrated.

Variable Types Emerging from Dynamic Data on Behaviours

Figure 5.1 presents three hypothetical types of variables encountered in population surveys on health which set out to estimate population behaviours. The word 'hypothetical' is used although the experience of collecting data over some time has shown that observed variables do correspond to these types. The questions of whether the variables in the population really behave in such a manner, and what portion of the observed phenomena is an artefact of total survey error, remain problematic and subject to further epistemological debate. Nonetheless, one may conceptualize at least three primary types of variables. Type A variables are relatively stable over time; show little variation over time; and possess a slope or incremental change over time which is largely observable and relatively constant, with little perturbation. Type B variables are less stable over time, but do illustrate some periodicity or

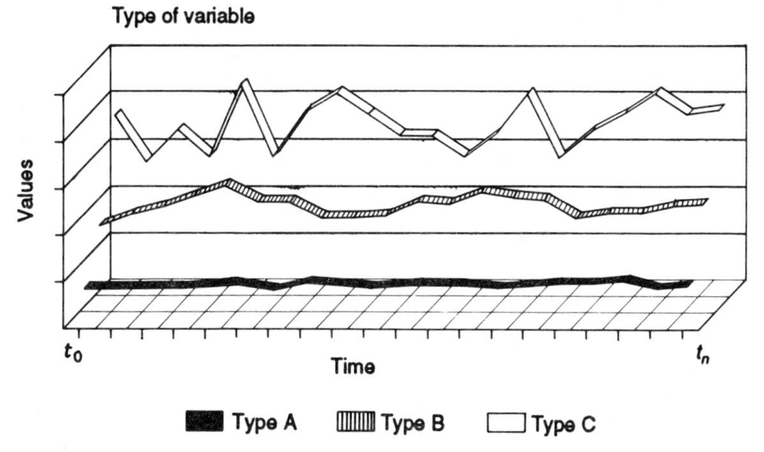

Figure 5.1 *Three types of variable: nature over time as expressed in population data*

regularity; may show some broad oscillatory behaviour and/or periods of reversals; and have a slope that varies. Type C variables are markedly unstable over time; are characterized by wide fluctuations; show marked rapid shifts in slope; and have quasi-regular patterns which are perhaps distinct over time, but catastrophic or chaotic behaviour is possible. Although these are hypothetical types of variable, survey researchers should recognize them in their data during either collection or analysis. Nevertheless, there is a problem for the survey researcher: if the focus is only on the analysis of cross-sectional data, at single points in time, these three hypothetical variables are difficult to distinguish from each other. That is, their true dynamics are masked.

There are different approaches for assessing the dynamic nature of behavioural variables over time (see the methods described by Nesselroade and Hershberger in Chapter 4). In order to observe the true dynamic nature of behavioural variables at the population level, one useful approach is to take the continuous data collecting approach using a rapid turn-around interviewing technique such as CATI provides. Table 5.2 shows the areas included in a CATI-based study in Scotland. The subject areas for inclusion are similar to those in other population health surveys concerned with health

Table 5.2 *The CATI questionnaire:*[1] *areas for questions and stability*

Survey item areas	Stability over time
Safety	High
Environment	Moderate
Exercise, fitness	Moderate
Eating behaviour	Low
Smoking and drinking	Moderate
Health practices	Low
Publicity on health	Low
AIDS-related AOB[2]	Low
Respondent details	High
Interviewer details	High

[1] The CATI questionnaire used to date has three components: (1) baseline questions which never change; (2) questions which remain relatively constant but are subject to changes in wording, response category etc.; and (3) questions which are introduced from time to time for experimental purposes or to develop a new subject area into the study. Over the period July 1987 to July 1992, the questionnaire was modified nine times, and thus there were nine versions of the instrument.

[2] AOB: attitudes, opinions, behaviours.

promotion and lifestyle which are carried out by telephone interview, such as the large-scale Canadian Health Promotion Survey (Rootman et al., 1989) and the behavioural risk factor surveys at the US Centers for Disease Control (Hogelin, 1988). In short, in terms of theoretical approach and questionnaire design there is little to distinguish it from other such surveys. Its unique feature is the continuous collection of data; thus one can begin to consider characteristics of the behavioural areas by their stability (and/or instability, periodicity etc.) over time. It should be emphasized that although most of the topic areas are standard, the inclusion of details about the interviewer's performance, and of a mini-questionnaire for the interviewer within the interview, is a particular strength of this data collection method. The addition of this component allows two very important considerations: (1) the role of the interviewer within a data collection error perspective; and (2) a more adequate analysis of cost and quality of the data collection process. These considerations place this survey within a total survey error perspective.

The estimates of stability over time on the right of Table 5.2 represent an estimate based on studying these topic areas and the variables/questions within the topics. Some are intuitively clear; for example seat-belt usage (safety subject) remains very stable in reporting, whereas eating practices are very unstable, undoubtedly reflecting the findings that behavioural change in diet is very volatile. Of course, any subject area is complex and is likely to have some more or less stable variables. Therefore, as an illustration, consider one area – AIDS-related attitudes, opinions and behaviours – in more detail.

Table 5.3 shows the area within the CATI-based continuous survey for question items on attitudes, opinions and behaviours related to AIDS. Many of the questions are identical or similar to questions asked in other population surveys on AIDS; one chief difference in this continuous survey is that these questions are embedded in a larger lifestyle and health (LAH) questionnaire. Thus the questions on AIDS enter after some general questions about publicity and health. Following a short introduction to the AIDS section the survey participant is asked a series of questions on opinions about AIDs. This is followed by some questions to ascertain the respondent's knowledge about AIDS. The questions related to blood (donation, transfusion etc.) are designed to complement questions on blood donation practice asked earlier in the questionnaire in the health practices section. The questions on AIDS as a problem relate to the respondent's perception of AIDS as a problem at different levels of social organization (community,

Table 5.3 *The CATI questionnaire(s): stability of AIDS attitudes, opinions and behaviours*

AIDS topic area	Stability over time
Publicity about AIDS	Variant
Opinions about AIDS	Variant
Knowledge about AIDS	Stable (+)
Blood and AIDS	Stable (+/−)
AIDS as a problem	Stable(−)
Talking about AIDS	Stable(−)
Change in behaviour	Stable(+)
Intention to change behaviour	Variant
Sexual practices	Stable(+)
Concern on risk of AIDS	Stable(−)

neighbourhood, country, area etc.). The questions on talking about AIDS ask about discussions with family and friends. The questions on changes in behaviour relate to change in sexual behaviour (use of condoms, fewer partners etc.); those on intentions to change parallel those on reported changes. The questions on actual sexual practice follow after a brief reminder of the anonymity of the survey (these questions are asked only of respondents aged 18–50).

As an example of stability observed in variables measured continuously, consider those related to knowledge. Five different items with 'correct' responses based on current medical opinion about AIDS make up an index of knowledge about AIDS. The questions are standard: whether one can get AIDS from kissing with exchange of saliva, from donating blood, from insect bites, from eating food prepared by someone with AIDS, and by using public toilets. But the stability and reliability of each of these items over time have given confidence in constructing a population knowledge index about AIDS. As can be seen in Figure 5.2, the resulting index is stable and possesses a stable increment of change over time.

In terms of its importance with respect to opinions and changing behaviours in relation to AIDS, talking about AIDS with others appears to be rather important. Nevertheless, reported talking about AIDS with other appears to be only moderately stable over time and is clearly less stable than knowledge about AIDS. Figure 5.3 shows the case for reported talking about AIDS with one's family in two cities in the sample. The pattern shows more reported discussion in the 'big city', but at the same time this pattern is more irregular than that in 'metrocity'. Coincidentally it is big city which has the larger AIDS problem. Figure 5.4 illustrates the smoothed trend line for each city, and this shows the slightly downward trend over time.

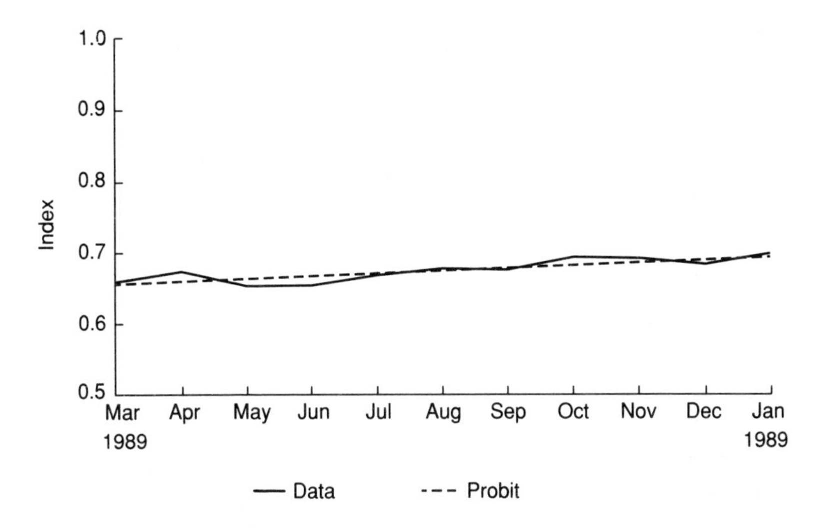

Figure 5.2 *AIDS knowledge over time: Scottish data with index constructed from five items which have been dichotomized (scale ranges from 0 to 1)*

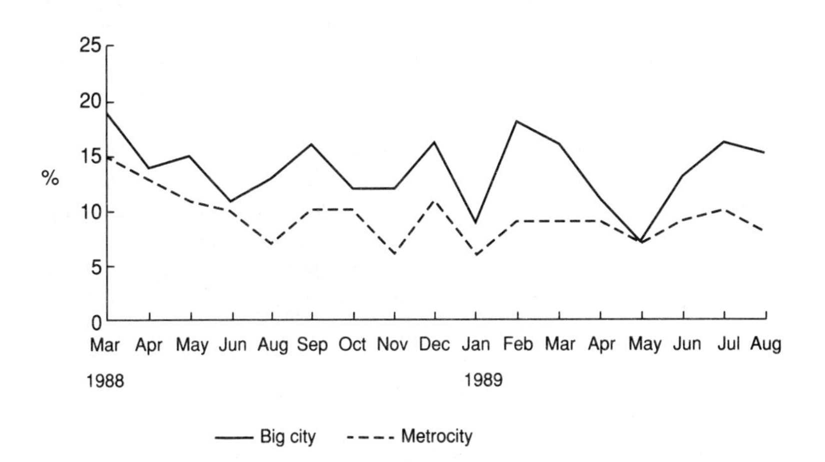

Figure 5.3 *Talk about AIDS with family (percentage of respondents saying 'often'). No data were collected for July 1988*

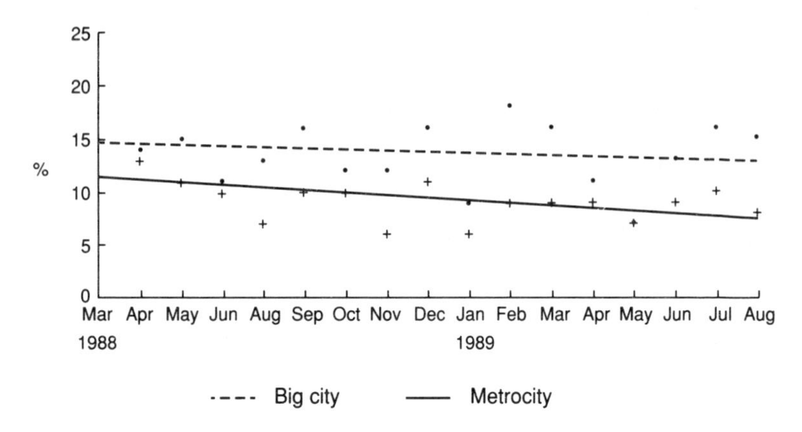

Figure 5.4 *Talk about AIDS with family, trend lines (percentage of respondents saying 'often'). No data were collected for July 1988*

Implications for Population Research

The major emphasis in this chapter has been on the value and importance of collecting data continuously. A number of issues follow from this data collection approach; three in particular should be emphasized.

First, data collection benefits from adopting a broader approach to the idea of error. In particular, a balance needs to be struck between statistical issues and sociological issues. This balance can be assisted by more attention being placed on the data collection process as a whole, taking the view that the instruments of data collection (CATI, interviewers, research teams, questionnaires etc.) are sources of error and explanation. Furthermore, one feasible and practical way to address the error problem, or elements of it, is to collect data continuously. Thus aspects of data collection such as question wording and interviewer effect take on meaning beyond simple error to be corrected statistically; they become part and parcel of the experimental nature of the data collection and may be seen as a characteristic of the instrument of data collection.

A second implication of the continuous data collection approach is to reveal some of the inadequacies of quasi-experimental designs in evaluation. Experimental designs for evaluation of interventions have dominated health promotion and sociomedical literature for many years. Underlying the approach is the idea of the population survey. The standard quasi-experimental (Cook and Campbell, 1979) approach is built around several assumptions: (1) a baseline survey; (2) one or more post-intervention surveys; (3) a control population; and (4) a well-circumscribed intervention. Numerous technical and practical issues underly each of these assumptions, for example that the baseline and subsequent surveys use a random sampling procedure; that the control population is not contaminated by the intervention being evaluated; and that the intervention operates without interference or augmentation from other possible interventions in the population. In reality, there are significant methodological problems with each of these assumptions, which have been elaborated in methodological literature of recent years. Despite these severe criticisms the quasi-experimental design has remained the standard approach in evaluation, notably in health education. In principle it is a rigorous and strong design; in practice it is problematic.

With the consideration of variables which are dynamic, that is concerned with behavioural change and process and necessarily containing a time component, static designs are inadequate – and the quasi-experimental design is static. Undoubtedly, part of the reason for maintaining such a rigorous and formal research design was the inability of population surveys, with their cumbersome data collection procedures, to collect and process data rapidly and in some kind of real time frame. New technology for interviewing, particularly CATI, has markedly altered the data collection process. The results of collecting data continuously with the new technology are only beginning to emerge, but this approach challenges the quasi-experimental approach and, therefore, seriously questions its use as the basis for evaluation of interventions. As illustration, consider Figures 5.5 and 5.6 which demonstrate some of the inherent pitfalls of a quasi-experimental approach.

Figure 5.5 shows a monthly plot of data collection continuously in a lifestyle and health survey with a section on AIDS. Data from two cities are shown in response to a question on whether or not the respondent has changed anything due to what they know about AIDS. As can be seen there are differences between the cities, and some differences, sometimes considerable, from month to month within the cities. Assume that a health promotion intervention regarding AIDS is planned for the month of October and the sponsors of the promotion desire an evaluation of the intervention. The classic experimental design would argue for a baseline survey prior to the intervention and then a post-intervention survey at some time after the intervention. An examination of the graph of the monthly cross-sectional data illustrates that the success or failure of the intervention, if changing something due to AIDS is an important outcome variable, is entirely dependent on what months

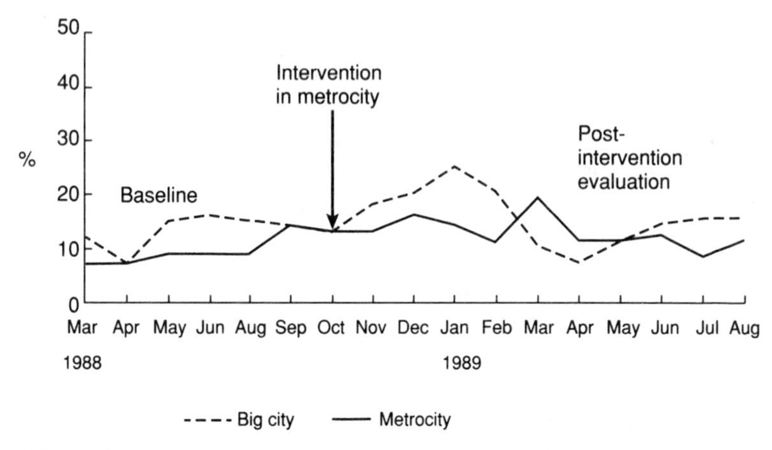

Figure 5.5 *Changed anything due to AIDS, hypothetical data (percentage of respondents saying 'yes'). No data were collected for July 1988*

are chosen for the baseline and the post-intervention survey. If one does not have such monthly cross-sectional data as shown here, the researcher is entirely in the dark as to what is happening in the population between periods of data collection. The data in Figure 5.5 show that following the intervention there was a considerable change in the population's response to the question, but that this change tapered off after some five months. To those planning the strategy of the intervention this is quite useful information, because it shows the possible waxing and waning of the intervention. Figure 5.6, which takes into account more completely the continuous nature of the data and looks at trends, shows that over time the respondents in both areas, big city and metrocity, were increasingly likely to report changing something, but the slight gap between the two cities has been decreasing since the intervention and the slope for metrocity is slightly steeper than that for big city. One might then conclude that an increase in the slope is a sign of relative success for the intervention strategy. Thus continuously collected data have allowed for an examination of the intervention which is impossible with a classical quasi-experimental design.

The third key issue concerns implications for data analysis. It is difficult to distinguish when data analysis begins. Traditionally, data collection might have been viewed as preparatory to analysis; that is, clean data, ready for analysis, implied that all the error had been reduced or taken out. Now it becomes clear that the data collection process cannot be easily separated from data analysis. In fact it could be argued that it is artificial to consider analysis as a separate

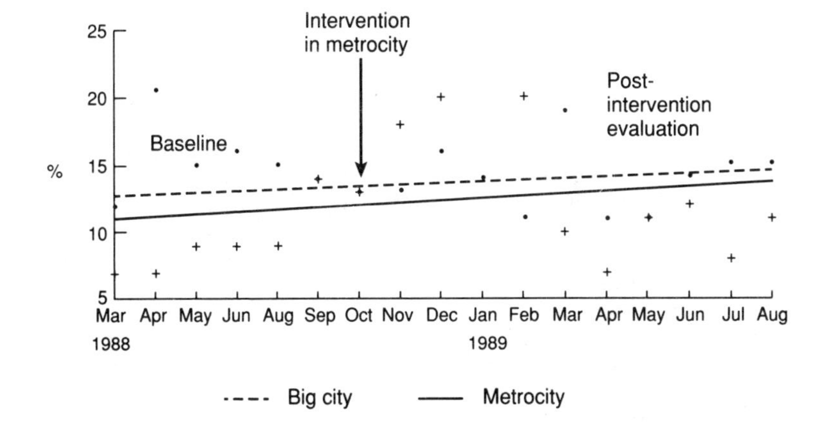

Figure 5.6 *Changed anything due to AIDS, hypothetical data, trend lines (percentage of respondents saying 'yes') No data were collected for July 1988*

stage of the research process. This implies a total survey approach which involves a type of feedback of data where later analyses begin to inform the interpretation of data analysed earlier. For example, as more data are collected over time, the unit of time which is appropriate for analysis (a day, a week, a month or a quarter) of the whole emerging data set becomes more clear in relation to the variation and stability of the variables being measured. Thus there is a synergistic effect of continuous data collection which can alter and shape decisions about analysis.

Other chapters in this book explore developing analytic approaches for complex population data. They argue that recent advances in computing and mathematical statistics need to be applied to large and complex data sets which are being and have been used in health research. This is an important point, but the possibility for the continuous collection of behavioural data at the population level using CATI introduces additional challenges for the analysis of complex data. While we have quite adequate analytic models for studying data collected over time (for example, time series analysis), these models are generally confined to a description of the data collected and do not provide an analysis of the interrelationships within the data where time is a variable. It remains a challenge for researchers to develop the analytic techniques to fully use the dynamic nature of continuously collected data.

Notes

1 Certainly in much of the writing on error the emphasis has been on sampling versus non-sampling error. Having said that, it is important to note the discrepancies which exist in the three areas of possible survey error, namely sampling, interviewing and questionnaire construction, in terms of the extent of the knowledge and available research. There is an enormous literature on sampling, and as a statistical issue it is well appreciated. However, much of the literature is mathematically sophisticated beyond the range of the social scientists; this is not to say that the issues involved cannot be questioned and expanded by a social science perspective. Indeed, statistical sampling, like any branch of a science, develops in a context which has many unscientific characteristics, and many considerations come into play in determining what is the acceptable meaning of sampling. Rituals and uncontested received wisdom play a role. However, quite sophisticated designs exist for coping with sampling issues. Nonetheless it is beginning to be appreciated that these sources of error are not necessarily independent one from another (Biemer et al., 1991).

2 Who are the participants in a survey? Certainly the classical notion is that the respondents are the participants. This is, in my opinion, a limited view of the survey process, particularly when one begins to consider the full ramifications of concepts as they are created by researchers, asked by interviewers, and answered by participants. Construct validity is an attempt to create an item which has some kind of true and equal meaning to researchers, interviewers and respondents. In that sense the three groups are coparticipants in the survey. The assumption that there is some kind of true fit among these three groups is largely untested.

3 All the examples where data are given come from the continuous survey on lifestyle and health carried out at RUHBC using CATI. The data collection began in July 1987; by April 1992 over 30,000 interviews had been completed. The data are collected on 18–60 year olds in households with telephones in the Glasgow, Edinburgh and London metropolitan areas. Sample selection is by a Waksberg (1978) random digit dialling (RDD) technique; 15 stand-alone IBM compatible microcomputers are used; the CATI is programmed using CASS software augmented by RUHBC programs; and data analysis is chiefly by SPSS. The staff consists of some 30 interviewers, five supervisor/interviewers, four research assistants, one statistician, one senior researcher and the principal investigator; additional support is provided by two secretaries and RUHBC research staff. Monthly data updates are published by RUHBC, in addition to reports of research and other publications. The research is funded by the Scottish Home and Health Department (SHHD), the Health Education Board of Scotland (HEBS) and the Economic and Social Research Council (ESRC).

4 There are also many insights which go into the rationale for a continuous data collection system. One is that one-shot, cross-sectional surveys are problematic even when well carried out. There are all the usual sources of survey error, and the added disadvantage of being able to correct for error only after the sampling and interview period is finished. Thus any adjustment for error relies almost entirely on post-survey statistical manipulations, missing the sociological concern with explanation. Anyone who has carried out a series of cross-sectional surveys on a population knows that the first cross-section is to a great extent a learning experience for those carrying out the research, in becoming familiar with the sampling strategy, settling in the interviewers and so on. The whole process is working well by the time the data collection period has ended. Nevertheless the problem is not necessarily solved by a longitudinal

design with a series because, depending on the intervals between surveys, each resurvey may require a new and massive effort for it to be carried out.

References

Biemer, B.P., Groves, R.M., Lyberg, L.E., Mathiowetz, N.A. and Sudman, S. (eds) (1991) *Measurement Errors in Surveys*. New York: Wiley.

Blalock, H.M. (1969) *Theory Construction*. Englewood Cliffs: Prentice Hall.

Coleman, J.S. (1964) *Introduction to Mathematical Sociology*. Glencoe, IL: Free Press.

Coleman, J.S. (1990) *Foundations of Social Theory*. Cambridge, MA: Harvard University Press.

Cook, T.D. and Campbell, D.T. (1979) *Quasi-Experimentation: Design and Analysis Issues for Field Settings*. Boston: Houghton-Mifflin.

Groves, R.M. (1989) *Survey Errors and Survey Costs*. New York: Wiley.

Hogelin, G. (1988) 'The behavioural risk factor surveys in the United States: 1981–1983', in R. Anderson, J.K. Davies, I. Kickbusch and D.V. McQueen (eds), *Health Behaviour Research and Health Promotion*. Oxford: Oxford University Press.

Lieberson, S. (1984) *Making it Count: the Improvement of Social Theory and Research*. University of California Press.

Nunnally, J.C. (1978) *Psychometric Theory*. New York: McGraw-Hill.

Rootman, I., Warren, R., Stephens, T. and Peters, L. (eds) (1989) *Canadian Health Promotion Survey*, technical report. Ottawa: Health and Welfare Canada.

RUHBC (1989) *Changing the Public Health*. Research Unit in Health and Behavioural Change, Edinburgh. Chichester: Wiley.

Steeh, C. (1981) 'Trends in nonresponse rates', *Public Opinion Quarterly*, 45: 40–57.

Steier, F. (ed.) (1991) *Research and Reflexivity*. London: Sage.

Tanur, J.M. (1983) 'Methods for large-scale surveys and experiments', in *Sociological Methodology: 1983–1984*. San Francisco: Jossey-Bass.

Tuma, N.B. and Hannan, M.T. (1984) *Social Dynamics: Models and Methods*. Orlando, FL: Academic Press.

6

Validation of Index Scales for Analysis of Survey Data: the Symptom Index

Svend Kreiner

Introduction

Index scales may be defined as functions of one or more separate items. This chapter considers summary scales counting the number of a specific kind of response to several related questions. Most of what will be said may however without difficulty be generalized to any kind of scale function, for example sums of scored responses, more complex functions or qualitative categorizations of response patterns.

The focus of the chapter will be on statistical procedures for validating scales, a problem that is usually dealt with in psychometric terms. A main point of view of this chapter is, however, that survey research is not psychometrics and that there are limits to the extent to which notions and techniques transfer from one domain or research to another. The substantive research problems dealt with in psychometrics are not the same as those that survey research tries to solve, even though they share certain statistical models and techniques. Validity in one context therefore does not automatically guarantee validity in another.

We illustrate these points of view with analyses conducted on symptom scales in the context of a population study of health and behaviour in Denmark. The investigation was designed to study complex relationships among social situational, behavioural and health variables, making it well suited for relating these issues to the purposes of this book. Details about the study and an overview of some of the findings are available elsewhere (Dean, 1986). Kreiner (1986) describes some aspects of the analysis based on recursive graphical models.

Interviews were conducted with a random sample of 450 persons between 20 and 80 years of age. The sample was representative of the age, sex and marital status distributions in Denmark at the time of the study.

The respondents were asked whether or not they had experienced any of the 37 different symptoms during the past six months. The original intention was to summarize the responses to the 37 symptoms into one single summary symptom index, counting the number of different symptoms experienced – a more or less standard procedure for a crude measure of general health status known to correlate closely to other measures of health. We refer to Jylhä et al. (1986) for a discussion and additional references. In the example in this chapter, we will consider the association between health measured by the symptom index and age, a problem that has received some attention in gerontological research. We stress however that the discussion here will be concerned with the methodological aspects of using the symptom index for this purpose.

Table 6.1 gives an overview of some of the more important study variables. The data set, quite typical for health surveys, is high dimensional. Most of the variables are discrete.

For simplicity of exposition the validity of the symptom index will be examined using a small subset of variables: a subscale defined by 12 of the original 37 items and three additional variables, namely self-rated health (SRH), age and gender. For this example we assume that the substantive research problem has to do with the age–health relationship and that other variables are included in the study in order to be able to assess possible confounding effects of these variables on the relationship.

Symptom indices and SRH scales have been used in many different studies to study the age–health relationship. Most of these report high correlation between symptom indices and SRH – a fact that is often taken as evidence of the validity of SRH scales (Fillenbaum, 1979). Relationships between age and symptom indices or SRH scales are inconsistent, despite the 'biological fact that health deteriorates with age' (Cockerham et al., 1983). Thornstam (1975) and Jylhä et al. (1986) report decreasing numbers of symptoms with age. Linn and Linn (1980), Murray et al. (1982) and Cockerham et al. (1983) find no interaction between age and number of symptoms. Thornstam (1975) and Linn and Linn (1980) find no association between age and self-reported health, Cockerham et al. (1983) report improving health with age, and Murray et al. (1982) and Jylhä et al. (1986) have evidence of the opposite relationship. The contradictory results underline the need for careful validation of symptom indices and other scales that purport to measure health.

Table 6.1 *The variables of the Danish health and self-care survey*

Self-reported health	
Very good	
Good	
Fair	
Poor	
Health items (symptom episodes)	
Cold	Back pain
Cough	Chest pain
Problems with nose and throat	Diaphragm pain
Fever	Arthritis
Headache	Overweight
Muscle pain	Haemorrhoids
Nausea	Rash
Stomach problems	Sleeplessness
Problems with digestion	Problems with mouth and gums
Constipation	Tiredness
No appetite	Problems with feet
Problems with eyes	Anxiety
Problems with ears	Nervousness
Difficulty in breathing	Depression
Dizziness, fainting	Allergies
Problems urinating	Asthma
Abdominal problems	High blood pressure
Sexual problems	Diabetes
	Coronary thrombosis
Other variables	
Psychological distress	Age
Attitudes	Marital status
Social network variables	Education
Stress	Income
Gender	Employment

Validity and Scalability in Psychometrics

Validity

The question of what defines a good instrument for measurement has been a matter of concern in the social sciences. Psychometrics focuses in this connection on two basic properties of empirical measurement:

Reliability concerns the extent to which a measuring procedure yields the same results on repeated trials.
Validity is a question of whether or not the instrument measures

what it is intended to measure, and whether or not there are limits to its use.

The notion of validity is the more subtle of the two requirements. It requires both theoretical constructs and theories linking constructs to each other and to empirically grounded indicators.

Psychometrics distinguishes between at least three main types of validity:

Content validity Do the observations truly sample the universe of situations linked to the theoretical construct?
Construct validity Is the measurement instrument linked to (nothing but) the correct attribute it is meant to measure?
Criteria validity Is the measurement instrument associated with other indicators linked to the theoretical construct?

Borhnstedt (1983) gives an excellent overview of the different notions of validity. Construct validity is identified as the overriding requirement, but construct validity and criteria validity to a certain extent overlap. Borhnstedt distinguishes between theoretical validity and criteria-related construct validity. Theoretical validity requires that the theoretical construct explains all of the covariation between different items of an index scale and between items and other variables. Criteria-related construct validity requires that no other variables are able to explain the relationship between the index scale on the one hand and another set of indicators or criteria on the other hand.

Scalability

In addition to validity, important technical aspects of measurement instruments must be considered: objectivity, adequacy, generalizability and reliability.

The conclusions drawn from the study have to be objective in the sense that they do not depend on more or less arbitrary decisions made during the study. Low-level (specific) objectivity refers to the study at hand and the available options for scaling. There may be a choice between several alternative scales defined by subsets of items from a larger 'theoretical' item bank without theoretical arguments favouring one specific version. Or we may have a choice between a long version of the index scale and a shorter, more practical one. Objectivity requires that results do not depend in any fundamental or systematic way on the choice made between alternative versions of the same scale.

Generalizability of an index scale refers to the problem of transferring knowledge about a scale's qualities in a specific context to a different study. It is common to stress that validation of a scale is always with respect to a given purpose and that generalization to completely different scenarios is not automatically given, but studies often occur where this concern seems to be forgotten. Once a scale has been reported as valid, the same scale is frequently used for all kinds of diverse purposes.

Adequacy of a measurement is a question of whether or not all of the available information has been summarized by the index function defining the scale. If not, then the scale is inadequate in the sense that in principle we are able to do better.

Finally, reliability is a question of the extent to which repeated measurements for the same subjects give the same results. An unreliable measurement is characterized by systematic bias between the first and the second measurement and/or by too much random noise.

The four different technical requirements – that scales are reliable, objective, adequate and generalizable – may be said to define a requirement of *scalability*. A good index scale has to be not only valid in the theoretical sense, but also *scalable* in the technical sense.

Local Independence and Unbiasedness

Psychometrics treats analysis of validity and scalability as strictly statistical problems. Certain assumptions are made concerning the structure and distribution of responses. The assumptions define a so-called measurement model, and the validation problems are treated as questions of estimating certain parameters and/or of checking the fit of these models to data. Theoretical constructs are represented in these models by latent unobservable variables. The requirements of construct validity are stated and checked in terms of conditional independence and conditional relationships. Items must be both mutually conditionally independent and conditionally independent of other manifest variables given the latent variable. Additionally, the index scale and criteria variables must be not only marginally but also conditionally dependent when the relationships are controlled for other manifest variables.

The condition that items are conditionally independent given the latent variable is what psychometricians understand as *local independence*. Conditional independence of items and other manifest variables is referred to as *unbiasedness* of items.

Subdisciplines of Psychometrics

Psychometrics embraces two major traditions, classical psychometrics and item response theory (IRT). Both disciplines are concerned with analysis of latent structure. Both disciplines distinguish between manifest responses on the one hand and latent variables or parameters on the other hand. Both disciplines attempt to express the manifest responses as probabilistic functions of the latent variables in terms of the conditional distribution of the manifest responses given the latent variables/parameters. The difference lies in the paradigms underlying the way the two branches of psychometrics tries to model these conditional distributions.

Classical Psychometrics

Classical psychometrics is based on a true score/measurement error paradigm expressing manifest responses (to items or scores) R in terms of expected values or true scores $T = E(R)$ and unbiased measurement errors:

$$R = T + E$$

Manifest responses may be items, subscales or composite tests. For a review of properties derived from the classical psychometric paradigm see Lord (1980: Chapter 1).

Expressing the manifest response as a sum of an expected true score and an unbiased error should not be regarded as an assumption. Any random variable can be expressed in this way. It is more like a declaration of intent in the sense that the natural next step is to try to model the true score and the error separately.

To do so, classical psychometrics introduces the following assumptions:

1 The true score is a linear function of the latent variable.
2 The latent variable (and therefore the true score) and the error are uncorrelated.
3 Latent variables and errors are normally distributed.

It follows from these apparently simple assumptions that classical psychometrics only has to be concerned with first- and second-order moments: means, variances and covariances/correlations. From these assumptions follow classical psychometrics, exploratory factor analyses and eventually so-called LISREL models for high-dimensional covariance structure.

Item Response Theory

The modelling paradigm of item response theory keeps the latent structure paradigm, but dispels with the explicit measurement error variables and linear structures. IRT models describe probabilities of specific manifest responses to items as general functions of item parameters and either person parameters or latent person *variables* characterizing the trait being measured by the scale in question. From these probabilities one may of course derive formulas for true scores and errors. The true score will however not in general be a linear function of a latent variable and the distribution of errors will typically depend on the values of the latent variables.

As an example, consider the so-called Rasch (1960/1980) model for binary items. Assume that item responses are coded 1 for a positive and 0 for a negative response. The model in this case expresses the probability of a positive response by person j on a given item i as a simple linear logistic function of unidimensional item and person parameters:

$$P(I_{ij}=1) = \exp(\alpha_i+\beta_j) / (1+\exp(\alpha_i+\beta_j)) \qquad (6.1)$$

The original Rasch model treated both item and person characteristics as parameters. Rasch made no assumptions concerning the variation of the person parameters within a given population. The model was in fact an explicit attempt to get rid of the routine assumptions of normally distributed traits that Rasch felt had contaminated psychometrics.

A latent variable model would however see β_j as the outcome of a latent variable B measuring a given trait in a specific population. The model (6.1) should in this case be restated in terms of the conditional distribution of item i given the value of this latent variable:

$$P(I_i=1 \mid B=b) = \exp(\alpha_i+b) / (1+\exp(\alpha_i+b)) \qquad (6.2)$$

The expected value of a 0/1 variable is equal to the probability of a positive response. The true score in this case is therefore equal to the probability (6.2), that is a logistic and not a linear function of the latent variable.

The error is defined as the difference between the observed outcome and the true score. That is, for a variable with two possible outcomes, with outcome 0 the error is $-\exp(\alpha_i+b) / (1+\exp(\alpha_i+b))$, and with outcome 1 the error is $1 / (1+\exp(\alpha_i+b))$.

The expected value of the error has to be zero whatever the value of the item parameter and the latent variable. In this sense the error may be said to be independent of the latent variable. The variance of the error, however, depends on the latent variable:

$$\exp(\alpha_i+b) / (1+\exp(\alpha_i+b))^2$$

Latent variables and errors therefore are not statistically independent in the Rasch model. It would make no sense to use the true-score/error decomposition of a Rasch model even though it is formally possible to do so.

Statistical models require some kind of simplification to be useful. The classical psychometric confidence in normal distributions therefore frequently reappears in IRT contexts – including the Rasch model – in connection with assumptions on the distribution of the latent variables, even though the models do not assume a linear relationship between the latent variable and the true score.

To replace the simplification inherent in the independent normally distributed errors of classical psychometric models, IRT introduces local independence, that is mutual conditional independence of items given the latent variable, as a fundamental assumption. This may at first look like a matter of convenience, because the possible number of unknown parameters in the models are reduced and the statistical procedures consequently simplified. As discussed above, however, local independence is closely related to theoretical construct validity. IRT models may therefore be regarded as a partial formalization of construct validity. Model checking of IRT models is one important step of a statistical test for construct validity. We refer to Rosenbaum (1989) for a complete discussion of the relationship between IRT models and construct validity.

Statistical Requirements

It is important to note at this point that there are no principal differences between the way classical psychometrics and item response theory see validity problems and especially construct validity. There are certain differences in the statistical procedures motivated by the different statistical models, but the overall aims are the same. It is in the assessment of scalability, the technical aspects of the scaling procedures, that the differences between the psychometric schools become apparent.

The overriding concern in classical psychometrics appears to be the question of reliability. The linear structure assumed by the classical psychometric models implies that optimal scales may be defined as simple linear functions (weighted means) of the scores associated with the separate items. The assumptions of normality of latent variables and errors ensure that objectivity and adequacy are almost automatically preserved. The only remaining technical problem consequently is the reliability, when the rather restrictive assumptions of classical psychometrics are met.

Things are not quite that simple for the general class of IRT models. Even though an IRT model may exist that adequately fits the data, it does not automatically follow that it is wise to calculate a summary scale in a given specific way. Replacement of the complete set of item responses by a summary scale is data reduction. It may imply loss of important information. We therefore have both to motivate a specific scaling procedure, and to justify its use by an analysis of the correspondence between empirical item responses and the assumptions that have to be met for objective and/or adequate scalability to be attained.

The *adequacy* of a given scaling procedure is best expressed in terms of statistical sufficiency. An adequate index has to be a statistically sufficient statistic for the unknown person parameter in the sense that the conditional distribution of item responses given the index scale does not depend in any way on these parameters. The corresponding concept in models with latent variables rather than latent parameters is conditional independence (Dawid, 1979). A scale is adequate if item responses are conditionally independent of latent variables given the summary index scale.

The *objectivity* of a procedure requires that conclusions drawn from the use of the scale only depend on aspects of the theoretical constructs (except possibly for pure random noise). Characteristics of the scaling procedure (for example, how and which items are drawn from a larger bank item) and the sampling of individuals for a calibration or validity study should not influence the results in any systematic way. Items should for instance be strongly interchangeable in the sense that conclusions must not depend on which specific items we use for the scale or the sequence in which they are presented to the respondent.

Properties of the Rasch Model

It turns out that objectivity and adequacy for locally independent binary items are one and the same thing, characterizing the so-called Rasch model (6.1). The Rasch model is the only IRT model for locally independent binary items where the raw score is a sufficient statistic for the unknown person parameters, and the only IRT model that gives specifically objective measurements. Testing the Rasch model is therefore equivalent to a test of theoretical construct validity and the adequacy of the scale.

Sufficiency implies that the conditional distribution of item responses given the raw score does not depend on the person parameters. This distribution – the conditional Rasch model – is easily derived from (6.1) or (6.2):

$$P(I_{ij}, \ldots, I_{kj} \mid \sum_i I_{ij}=s) = \exp\left(\sum_i I_{ij}\alpha_i\right) / \Gamma_s(\alpha) \qquad (6.3)$$

where

$$\Gamma_s(\alpha) = \sum_{I_i} \ldots \sum_{I_k} \exp\left(\sum_i I_i\alpha_i\right), \quad I_i + \ldots + I_k = s$$

We refer to Rasch (1966) and Andersen (1977) for arguments

leading from either objectivity or sufficiency to characterizations of the Rasch model.

Construct validity implies local independence of items. This requirement is satisfied by several different item response models. The important point to emphasize here is that the Rasch model is the only IRT model for binary items that also meets the dual requirements of objectivity and adequacy. The Rasch model may in this sense be said to be the necessary and sufficient condition for scalability within the general class of item response models.

Several graphical and numerical techniques have been suggested for tests of fit of the Rasch model (Andersen, 1980; Gustafsson, 1980; Andrich, 1988). The best and most reliable are those that test the fit of the conditional Rasch model. It is therefore of interest to note that the conditional Rasch model appears naturally from the latent variable model (6.2), where the person parameters are replaced by a latent *variable*, and where the sufficiency condition has to be replaced by conditional independence between the item responses and the latent variable given the raw score.

There are two conclusions to be drawn from this observation. First, we are permitted to use precisely the same techniques in two similar but distinct contexts – with fixed person parameters and with latent random variables. A third context will appear later in this paper. Second, we only have indirect validation of either the classical Rasch model or the corresponding model with latent variables. No statistical test of fit can tell us whether the first or the second model is the more appropriate. We are talking about completely different modelling paradigms, the appropriateness of which depends on the purpose of the statistical analysis.

The transfer of a specific statistical technique between two different models (in this case the test of fit of the conditional Rasch model) is an example of scale generalizability. Given the similar structure of the two models, we have perhaps no reason to be surprised, but we should remember that other techniques for testing the Rasch model based on the unconditional distributions do not transfer. Generalizability therefore is not trivial; it is not automatically attained.

The missing generalizability suggests that validity is not an absolute property of a scale. Validity inevitably raises the question: valid in which frame of reference and for what purpose? Different validation procedures build upon different statistical models. The question raised here is whether or not an analysis motivated by a specific statistical model makes sense at all as seen from a different model. We have seen that this is the case for certain procedures based on the conditional Rasch model but not necessarily for other procedures. The question therefore remains for other types of models and other types of validation procedures: how far do these procedures reach?

Psychometric Validation of the Symptom Index

This section gives first a short overview of some of the results obtained during the validation of the symptom index, and secondly the results concerning the relationship between age and health as measured by the index.

Table 6.2 defines the symptom index and displays the marginal distributions for the 450 cases of the Danish survey of health and self care.

Table 6.3 shows the association between the symptom index and self-reported health. The product moment correlation between these variables was highly significant ($r = 0.28$). The product moment correlation may however not be an appropriate statistic for

Table 6.2 *The 12 items included in the symptom index*

Items

Cough	Nose and throat
Muscle pain	Fever
Eyes	Stomach
Dizziness, fainting	Indigestion
Back pain	Rash
Chest pain	Mouth and gums

Score distribution

Score	Count	%	Cum.
0	180	40.0	40.0
1	140	31.1	71.1
2	73	16.2	87.3
3	43	9.6	96.9
4	10	2.2	99.1
5	2	0.4	99.5
6	1	0.2	99.7
7			
8			
9			
10			
11	1	0.2	99.9
12			
Total	450	99.9	

Table 6.3 *Distribution of symptom index by self-reported health*

SRH	Symptom score 0 (%)	1 (%)	2 (%)	3–12 (%)	Total *n*
Very good	48.7	29.1	13.9	8.2	158
Good	44.0	34.0	11.3	10.7	150
Fair	30.9	32.7	24.5	11.8	110
Poor	7.4	14.8	25.9	51.9	27

$\chi^2 = 60.8$ d.f. = 9 $p = 0.000$ gamma = 0.292 $p = 0.000$

Table 6.4 *Observed versus expected counts of nose and throat problems for different score groups*

Symptom score	*N*	Observed	Expected
1	140	23	13
2	73	12	16
3	43	12	14
4	10	3	4
5	2	1	1
6	1	0	1
11	1	1	1
4–11	14	5	7

highly skewed discrete data. We therefore calculated Goodman-Kruskal's gamma for Table 6.3, which also provided very strong evidence of interaction. We conclude that the symptom index is criteria valid to a reasonably high degree.

Construct validity and scalability were investigated from the point of view of the classical Rasch model with latent person parameters. The check of the model was performed as a check of the conditional Rasch model for item responses given raw scores. Andersen's (1980) conditional likelihood ratio test comparing item parameters in different score groups was used for a general test of fit of the model, while several different methods (graphical procedures and analysis of residuals) were used to assess heterogeneity of specific items and local independence of items.

The general fit of the conditional Rasch model was very satisfactory, with signs of specific problems few and unsystematic. Andersen's conditional likelihood ratio gave 31.4 with 22 degrees of freedom ($p = 0.09$).

Table 6.5 *Distribution of symptom index by age*

Age	Symptom score 0 (%)	1 (%)	2 (%)	3–12 (%)	Total n
20–40	42.1	32.7	15.3	9.9	202
41–55	36.6	30.4	17.4	15.5	161
56+	41.4	28.7	16.1	13.8	87
Total	40.0	31.1	16.2	12.7	450

$\chi^2 = 3.6$ d.f. $= 6$ $p = 0.72$ gamma $= 0.06$ $p = 0.30$

Table 6.4 shows the correspondence between observed and expected counts for nose and throat problems in different score groups, the only item providing the slightest evidence against the conditional Rasch model. The fit is less than perfect for cases with only one symptom. As no other evidence was found, however, we feel justified in concluding that the symptom index is both construct valid and adequate.

The final analysis considers the dependence of the symptom index on age and gender. No evidence was found against conditional independence of symptom index and gender given age. The problem therefore reduces to an analysis of the marginal Table 6.5, where no evidence against independence of age and symptom index is to be found. The number of symptoms is clearly not correlated with age.

Logic of Statistical Modelling

The validation reported in the previous section is more or less routine. We have looked at the symptom index from several different viewpoints and in no cases found any noteworthy problems. The acceptance of the Rasch model is especially promising, because the requirements underlying the model are very demanding.

There are, nevertheless, problems. To see this one must consider the validation procedure from a strictly statistical point of view. Figure 6.1 illustrates the situation. The findings presented above come from three completely different statistical analyses, each with its own aims and each based on three quite different models.

Criteria validity was established by a marginal model describing the association between self-reported health and the symptom index. To interpret the correlation coefficients as coefficients of validity we have to take a classical psychometric viewpoint assuming

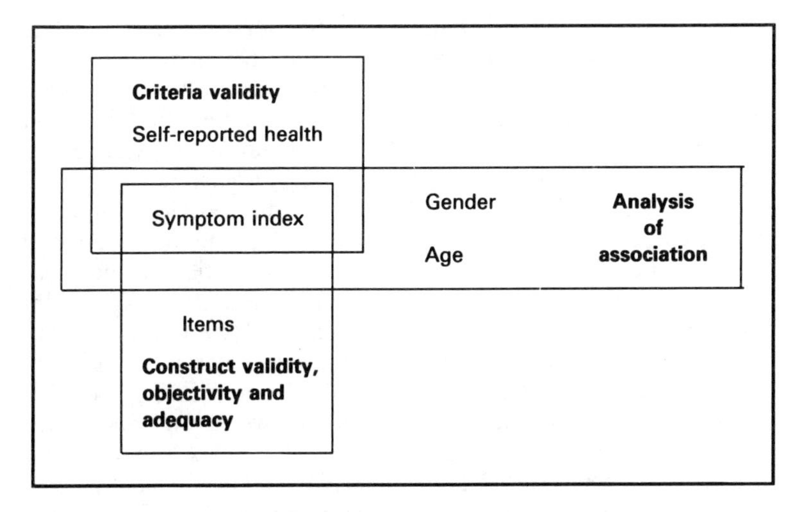

Figure 6.1 *Schematic representation of the three frames of inference for the symptom index*

a general latent health variable underlying the manifest scores of the symptom index.

Construct validity, objectivity and adequacy are ensured by the fit of the Rasch model. This is a very strong result, and apparently precisely the result needed to justify in statistical terms the use of the symptom index for the analysis.

Finally we have the analysis of association between health, gender and age. The model we use here is a standard log-linear or graphical model appropriate for analysis of qualitative data.

Taken separately, there is nothing wrong with any of these analyses (although certain aspects of the analysis as presented here of course could be improved). We are using standards methods based on standard modelling paradigms to address standard problems.

Taken together, however, logical problems arise from this work. Note that the final analysis based on the log-linear model is the definitive analysis answering the substantive research questions. The sole purpose of the initial validation of the symptom index was to justify the use of the symptom index used in this final specific analysis.

The log-linear model is a model containing only manifest variables. The following questions therefore immediately spring to mind. Does it make sense *first* to fit models containing latent variables or parameters, and *then* to proceed to an analysis based on a model that has nothing at all to do with latent structure? Can we argue that the results of the first analyses are the vindication of the use of the symptom index for the definitive analysis? The symptom index is objective and adequate as seen from a point of view defined by a latent parameter: is it therefore also automatically objective and adequate in a model containing nothing but manifest variables?

The answer is no. These models have nothing at all in common. Validity from the point of view of one model cannot be assumed to have any bearing on analyses from the point of view of the other models. We refer to a recent discussion of these issues in a latent variable modelling context by Fornell and Yi (1992), but note that the problem is quite general. It appears in any statistical context where data are analysed by more than one statistical model. Therefore to proceed we have to choose between two options. We may reconsider the properties of the symptom index from the point of view of the type of model intended for the definitive analysis, that is from the point of view of a log-linear graphical model for manifest variables. Or we have to replace this model with a latent structure model based on either classical psychometric or IRT paradigms.

The next section considers the first of the two scenarios for two reasons. First, validation of scales from the viewpoint of the statistical models without latent structure has not been dealt with in depth before. Secondly – and more importantly – we do not think that a specific validation technique should determine the complete frame of inference for the analysis. Statistical techniques should follow from statistical models, not the other way round.

Validation without Latent Structure

The problems with the incompatible procedures for validation of scales and statistical analysis of association have to do with an implicit three-step strategy for the statistical analysis: (1) validation of scales, (2) choice of a statistical frame of inference, and (3) analysis of association.

The choice of validation procedures was routinely regarded as a matter of psychometric technique, while the choice of a statistical model for the analysis of the health–age association in this case had a bearing only on the three-dimensional data set containing gender, age and symptom index. Arguments motivating the different validation techniques disclose incongruities and suggest that there are logical problems. To get around these problems it is necessary to embark on the statistical analysis by defining a common frame of inference, a statistical model, for the complete set of variables including items of the symptom index and self-related health.

A Graphical Frame of Inference for Validation of Index Scales

The initial frame of inference for the analysis of the age–health association contains 16 variables, namely 12 items, a suggested index scale *S*, self-reported health status *H*, gender *X* and age *Y*. The analytic problem is simplified if we choose the general class of graphical models for the initial frame of inference. Graphical models are a general family of models assuming only pairwise conditional independence of variables. We may later refine the model by imposing additional assumptions on the data, but the family of graphical models is admirably suited as a starting point for analysis of association in high-dimensional contexts. Conditional independence is a part of basic probability theory. Using the family of graphical models as the initial frame of inference therefore does not require questionable assumptions about the structure of data. Conditional independence is common to all types of multi-dimensional model.

There are at least two tangible advantages of using graphical models as a starting point. First, the assessment of the scale is simplified considerably because we are able to restate many of the requirements of the scale in terms of the independence graphs associated with the models. Secondly, decompositions of the likelihoods – which may be read directly off the independence graphs – define collapsibility properties that justify the analysis of data in marginal data sets. Decompositions imply data reduction of the kind we talked about in connection with the notion of the adequacy of scales.

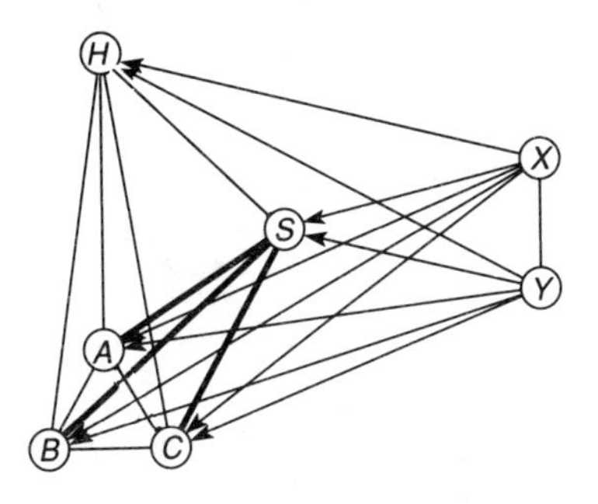

Figure 6.2 *The initial frame of inference. No assumptions are made concerning interaction or no interaction between variables,* S *is defined as a function of* A, B *and* C, *for which reason there is a strong interaction between these variables: this is indicated by the thick edges*

Figures 6.2–6.7 describe the situation with three items A, B and C, a summary scale S, self-reported health H and two exogenous variables X and Y. These graphs presume a recursive structure with the exogenous variables as explanatory variables, but the discussion generalizes without problems to situations with any number of prior and concurrent exogenous variables. The initial frame of inference is shown in Figure 6.2

Adequacy and Unbiasedness

We intend to use S as a summary scale replacing the original items A, B and C. The qualities of a good scale were discussed earlier. In the analysis of high-dimensional survey data, data reduction is imperative and may be the main reason why a scale is needed. Adequacy, in the sense that the scale summarizes all the available information contained in a set of item responses, therefore seems to be a central requirement.

The natural operationalization of this requirement is that items are conditionally independent of all other variables given the index:

$$ABC \perp HXY \mid S \tag{6.4a}$$

Relation (6.4a) is attained by the stronger requirement that

> any item is conditionally independent of any exogenous variable given the rest of the variables (for example, that $A \perp X \mid BCHYS$, that $B \perp X \mid ACHYS$ etc.) (6.4b)

Requirement (6.4b) defines the graphical model shown in Figure 6.3. This model implies that under no conditions (definable by the variables of our model) will there be any association between any item and any exogenous variable when we control for the value of the symptom index. These assumptions imply the crucial requirement defining adequacy: collapsibility onto the $HSXY$ variables.

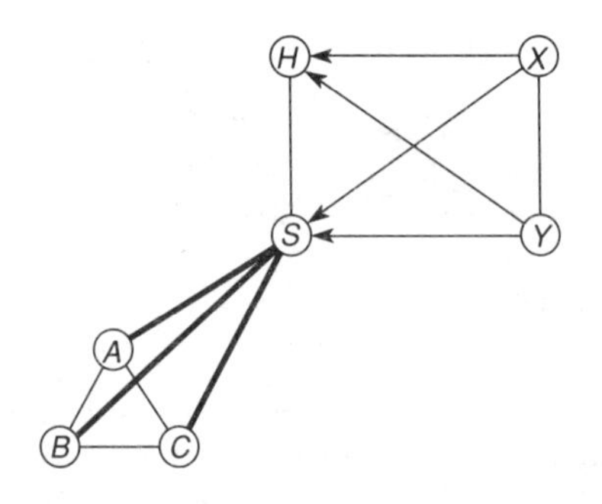

Figure 6.3 *Independence graph assuming no interaction between items and exogenous variables given index* S

Estimates of parameters describing the *HXY* interactions and tests for no interaction between *H* and *XY* calculated for the marginal *HSXY* data set are the same as estimates and test statistics calculated for the complete data set. Nothing at all of interest is lost by only considering the four *HSXY* variables if requirement (6.4b) is met.

Interesting and useful properties follow immediately from the model, Figure 6.3, and the so-called separation theorem of graphical models (Whittaker, 1990):

$$\text{any item} \perp \text{any exogenous variable} \mid \text{index} \qquad (6.5a)$$
$$\text{any item} \perp \text{self-reported health} \mid \text{index} \qquad (6.5b)$$

Properties (6.5a) and (6.5b) correspond exactly to one definition of *unbiased items* given in the psychometric literature:

> An item is considered unbiased when all persons at a given ability level have an equal probability of correctly answering an item regardless of their group membership. (Osterlind, 1983: 38)

The basic requirement of a good scale thus focuses on one of the more peripheral concepts from psychometric theory. Properties (6.5a) and (6.5b) are very easily checked using standard programs for analysis of contingency tables. No special techniques are required.

Noticing that (6.5a) and (6.5b) do not imply (6.4b), we may refer to (6.4b) as a requirement of *strongly unbiased items*. This strengthening of a well-known concept is all we need from psychometrics in order to justify the use of a scale. We notice also that no assumption has been made at all about the types of item or the function defining the scale. The assumptions about conditional independence and collapsibility on functions of items are completely general. They apply to all types of unidimensional or multidimensional scales.

Criteria Validity

Criteria validity requires that the scale is closely associated with other measurements based on the same underlying concept. The natural way to introduce criteria validity in a multidimensional framework is however somewhat stronger than a requirement of a high marginal correlation between the scale and the criteria. Strong criteria validity requires that the relationship between the index and the criteria cannot be explained by any of the remaining variables. That conditioning with respect to all variables in the study will not result in conditional independence between symptom index and self-reported health status. This situation is illustrated in Figure 6.4, where the edge between *H* and *S* has been emphasized to stress the strong inevitable interaction between these variables.

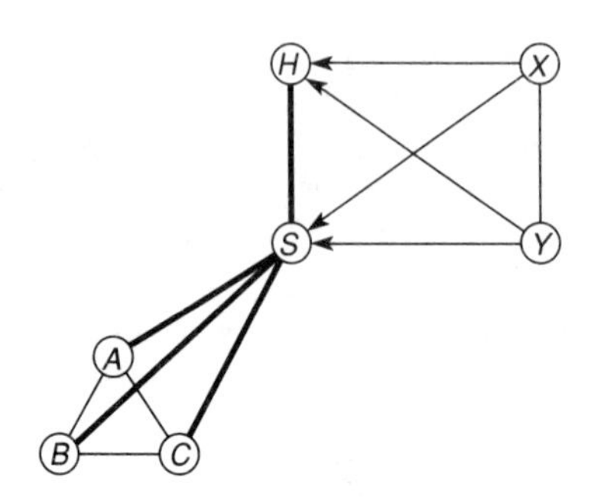

Figure 6.4 *Independence graph assuming no interaction between items and exogenous variables given index* S. *The interaction between index and self-reported health status has been emphasized*

The requirements on correlation coefficients defined by classical psychometrics have here been turned into requirements on non-vanishing *partial* correlations. A non-vanishing partial correlation coefficient implies *strong criteria validity*.

Choosing the Better of Two Scales

The next consideration has to do with whether or not the criteria variable should be excluded from the final analysis, that is whether or not the symptom index or the SRH variable is the better scale for analysis of the association between health and other variables. Again the answer is quite simple in graphical terms, referring to both conditional independence and collapsibility.

The problem of choosing the best scale is related to the problem motivating interest in the reliability of classical psychometrics. The less random noise inherent in a scale, the better. Or, phrased positively, the more relevant information contained in a scale, the better.

From this point of view, the answer to the above question is simple. The suggested scale is better than the criteria variable if all information contained in the criteria is also contained in the scale: in other words, if the criteria and the exogenous variables are conditionally independent given the scale.

The symptom index is therefore a better scale than the self-rated health, if the self-rated health H is conditional independent of all other variables given the scale:

$$H \perp XY \mid S \qquad (6.6a)$$

Relation (6.6a) is implied by the stronger requirements

$$H \perp X \mid YS \qquad (6.6b)$$

$$H \perp Y \mid XS \qquad (6.6c)$$

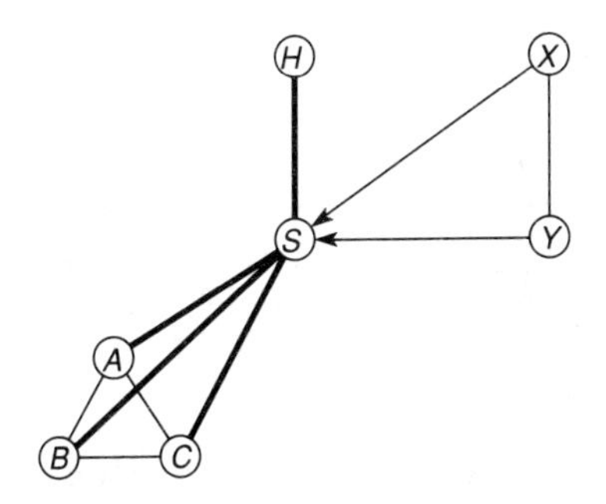

Figure 6.5 *Independence graph assuming no interaction between items and exogenous variables* H *and between the criteria and exogenous variables*

characterizing the graphical model defined by Figure 6.5. Notice that criteria validity under the conditions defined by Figure 6.5 turns into a requirement of non-vanishing marginal correlations.

Figure 6.5 defines a situation that permits us to use nothing but the symptom index as the measure of health. Under conditions (6.4b), (6.5a) and (6.5b) the problem reduces to the three-dimensional analysis of the *SXY* interaction reported earlier.

A check of the adequacy of a given scale should of course include a check that the criteria variable is not a better scale than the suggested scale in the sense defined by (6.6b) and (6.6c). If neither of the measures is better than the other, we have a situation related to the notion of discriminant validity, implying that both the scale and the criteria should be included in the analysis.

Objectivity and Local Independence

Apart from the natural tests for unbiased items no psychometric techniques have appeared yet, even though the basic problems to a certain degree at least are shared by psychometrics and the requirements for scaling in multidimensional statistical contexts.

Standard techniques reappear however when we consider the problem of objectivity. This problem becomes unavoidable the moment we consider scales defined by a more or less haphazard sample of items from a larger item bank. What one should require in this situation is that conclusions drawn from the use of a scale should be the same (except of course for purely random noise) as the conclusion we would draw from any other scale defined by a subset of items from our item bank.

Assume that the conditional distribution of items I, given exogenous variables X, depends on a set of interaction parameters $\beta(x)$:

$$P(I = i \mid X = x = f(i, \beta(x)) \qquad (6.7)$$

where both I and X are multidimensional vectors.

It follows directly from the requirement of adequacy (strongly unbiased items) that the summary index scale and the vector of exogenous variables ($S = \Sigma I_j$, X) comprise a statistically sufficient statistic for the β parameters with conditional distribution of S given X depending on β:

$$P(S = s \mid X = x) = g(s, \beta(x)) \qquad (6.8)$$

Objectivity requires that the interaction parameters are the same for all versions of the scale even though both g and f functions may be different. Items should be *exchangeable*: a new scale defined by exclusion of some items and inclusion of others should not affect the interaction parameters of interest.

Special cases of such interchangeable scales would of course be scales defined by separate items. It follows therefore that the number of interaction parameters that we use to describe the interaction between health and other variables should never be larger than the number of parameters in models for separate items instead of scales.

Arguing from cases with scales defined as the sum of two items, it follows from the sufficiency requirement that

> items must be conditionally independent of each other given all other variables (6.9)

and that the conditional distribution of separate binary items must follow a logistic regression model with an interaction parameter $\beta(x)$ common to all items:

$$P(I_j = 1 \mid \mathrm{X} = \mathrm{x}) = \exp(\alpha_j + \beta(x)) / (1 + \exp(\alpha_j + \beta(x))) \qquad (6.10)$$

The structure defined by (6.9) is shown in Figure 6.6, but we notice that with (6.10) we have abandoned the class of strictly graphical models. Objectivity imposes structure beyond what we can express in terms of nothing but conditional independence.

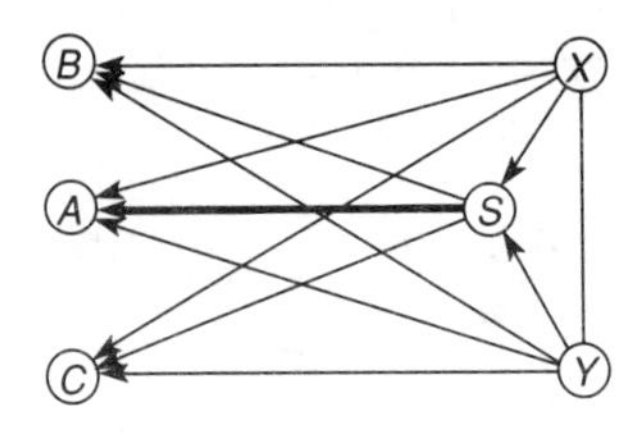

Figure 6.6 *Independence graph assuming conditionally independent items*

If (6.10) holds for all items and if items are conditionally independent as defined by Figure 6.6, then the raw score $S=\Sigma I_j$ and the exogenous variables are sufficient for the β parameters. All requirements for good scales discussed so far are met, and the interaction parameter that we may estimate will be the same whatever subscale we choose for our analysis. (The estimates will not be the same, of course, but differences between estimates from different subscales will be due to pure random noise.)

We notice that (6.9) is analogous to the psychometric requirement of local independence, while the logistic model (6.10) of course is almost a Rasch model. It is also of interest to see that local independence (6.9) appears as a consequence of objectivity requirements, whereas in psychometrics it is derived from the requirements of construct validity.

Model Checking

From the point of view of model checking we have several important results. It is easy to see that the conditional distribution of items given the raw score is a conditional Rasch model. Item analysis based on the conditional Rasch distribution is therefore also called for in connection with this model. Item analysis by the unconditional Rasch distribution, on the other hand, is of no consequence here.

Notice also that items from a subscale should be conditionally independent of other items given the subscale, as illustrated in Figure 6.7. This property was used by Tjur (1982) considering subscales with two items, but may be easily generalized to (sub)-scales with more than two items.

Finally we notice that the conditional distribution of the summary index scale given the exogenous variables must follow a so-called power series regression model:

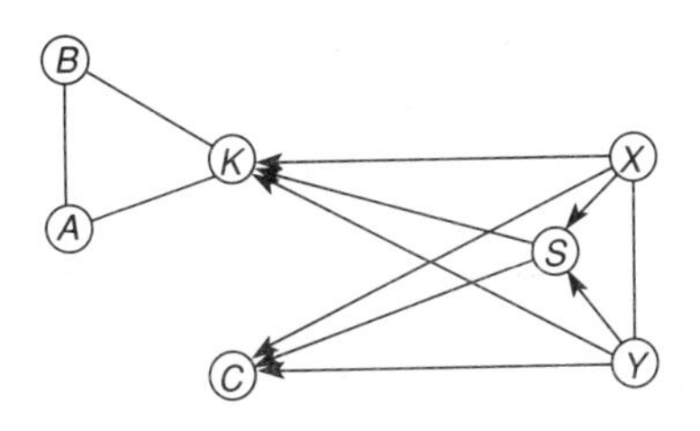

Figure 6.7 *The independence graph of the model with the subscale defined by* K = A+ B

$$P(S = s \mid X = x) = \tau(x)^s\Theta_s/\Sigma \qquad (6.11)$$

where Θ are so-called score parameters with values determined by the item parameters, $\tau = \exp(\beta)$ and Σ is a normalizing constant. Relation (6.11) may be expressed as a log-linear model, in which case it is seen to correspond to a standard model for ordinal categories. If probabilities of positive responses to separate items are small, the conditional distribution of scores given exogenous variables may be approximated by Poisson distributions. Objectivity thus implies a very simple structure that may be utilized in the statistical analysis of association between the scale and exogenous variables.

The Inadequacy of the Symptom Index

The analysis of the properties of the symptom index by graphical log-linear models is straightforward given the considerations of the previous section. The first concern is item bias with respect to age, because this is the primary variable of interest, and to SRH and gender. Analysis of item bias implies tests for conditional independence between items and exogenous variables in three-way tables with the total score as conditioning variable. This is a very simple type of analysis for which no specialized programs are needed. It nevertheless addresses the problems of the adequacy of the scale in a very direct way, and usually exposes most of the problems that we may find using more specialized and demanding techniques for item analysis.

Evidence of item bias with respect to age is found for several

Table 6.6 *Item bias: muscle pain and age*

Symptom score	Age	Muscle pain (%)	*N*
1	<40	13.6	66
	40–59	36.7	49
	60–	44.0	25
2	<40	32.3	31
	40–59	67.9	28
	60–	42.9	14
3–12	<40	55.0	20
	40–59	56.0	25
	60–	83.3	12
$\chi^2 = 22.7$ d.f. $= 6$ $p = 0.001$		partial gamma $= 0.43$ $p = 0.000$	

Table 6.7 *Item bias of stomach problems with respect to age*

Symptom score	Age	Stomach problems (%)	*N*
1	<40	4.5	66
	40–59	2.0	49
	60–	0.0	25
2	<40	19.4	31
	40–59	3.6	28
	60–	7.1	14
3–12	<40	20.0	20
	40–59	20.0	25
	60–	8.3	12

$\chi^2 = 6.4$ d.f. $= 6$ $p = 0.38$ partial gamma $= -0.45$ $p = 0.014$

Table 6.8 *Tests for item bias with respect to age*

Symptom	χ^2	d.f.	*p*	Gamma	*p*
Muscle pain	22.7	6	0.001	+0.43	0.000
Dizziness	6.5	6	0.37	+0.33	0.06
Nose and throat	5.1	6	0.52	−0.23	0.04
Fever	9.6	6	0.14	−0.77	0.002
Stomach	6.4	6	0.38	−0.45	0.014
Rash	7.8	6	0.26	−0.26	0.04
Mouth and gums	7.3	6	0.29	−0.40	0.01

items. Tables 6.6 and 6.7 show two of the strongest cases. We have increasing frequency of muscle pain and decreasing frequency of stomach problems with age for all score groups (with scores 3–12 collapsed into one group). In both cases significant evidence was disclosed by Davis's (1967) partial coefficient for Goodman-Kruskal's gamma. Table 6.8 shows that the problem with item bias is not restricted to these two items. Significant item bias is found for seven of the twelve items, suggesting very serious problems for the symptom index. No item bias was found with respect to gender and SRH. The bias problem is apparently a specific age phenomenon.

For completeness we also give the results of the analysis based on the conditional Rasch model. The initial analysis of the symptom index by the Rasch model established that there was no evidence of heterogeneity of items across different score groups. Likelihood ratio tests comparing estimates of item parameters for men and women, for persons with different experience of general health and for different age groups are shown in Table 6.9. The results

Table 6.9 *Test for homogeneity with respect to exogenous variables in the conditional Rasch model*

Exogenous variable	Likelihood ratio	d.f.	p
Gender	11.6	11	0.40
Self-reported health	36.9	33	0.29
Age	50.8	22	0.0004

Table 6.10 *Frequency of symptoms (per cent) in different age groups*

Symptom/episode	Age <40	Age 40–59	Age 60–
Cough	5.1	7.8	11.8
Muscle pain	25.6	50.0	52.9
Eyes	12.8	15.7	21.6
Dizziness	6.8	7.8	17.7
Back pain	23.9	31.4	19.6
Chest pain	4.3	8.8	7.8
Nose and throat	22.2	18.6	13.7
Fever	8.6	3.9	0.0[1]
Stomach	11.1	6.9	3.9
Digestion	12.0	6.9	13.7
Rash	24.8	14.7	15.7
Mouth and gums	13.7	11.8	5.9

[1] Significant evidence against marginal independence of age and symptom.

correspond closely to the results of the analysis of item bias. We have strong evidence of homogeneity across age groups, but no evidence at all of heterogeneity with respect to the other variables.

The results warrant a closer look at the age–symptom relationships. The marginal relationships are displayed by Table 6.10. The symptoms may be roughly partitioned into two equal groups characterized by respectively increasing and decreasing frequencies with age. Significant evidence of marginal age–symptom associations was however only found for muscle pain, dizziness and fever.

The evidence in Table 6.10 (together with other results not shown here) suggests that we at least consider two different scales, A and B, as shown in Table 6.11. The analysis of the adequacy of these scales along the same lines as above for the total symptom index disclosed no problems at all: no item bias, no heterogeneity across age groups, nothing at all in fact to be concerned about.

Table 6.11 *Homogeneous subscales*

Index A	Index B
Cough	Nose and throat
Muscle pain	Fever
Eyes	Stomach
Dizziness	Indigestion
Back pain	Rash
Chest pain	Mouth and gums

Table 6.12 *Marginal and partial correlations between health variables and age*

	Gamma coefficients			
Variables	Marginal	*p*	Partial	*p*
Indices A and B	0.25	0.001	0.29	0.001
Index A and SRH	0.30	0.000	0.17	0.016
Index B and SRH	0.25	0.000	0.25	0.002
Index A and age	0.27	0.000	0.22	0.003
Index B and age	−0.24	0.001	−0.38	0.000
SRH and age	0.26	0.000	0.20	0.004

It only remains to report on the analysis of association between symptom indices, SRH, gender and age. No evidence was found of any kind of association between gender and the other four variables. Symptom indices, SRH and age, on the other hand, were strongly associated. Table 6.12 displays Goodman-Kruskal's gamma coefficients for the marginal relationships and partial gamma coefficients calculated in the four-way marginal table collapsed across gender, but containing the other four variables.

To the extent that the three health variables may validate each other we have strong criteria valid scales. Symptom indices and SRH are strongly positively correlated. We also have divergent validity with respect to age as all partial gamma coefficients between age and health variables are highly significant. All three variables are needed then for a complete description of the age–health association.

The most noteworthy result, however, is the negative gamma coefficient between symptom index B and age. While both SRH and index A suggest deteriorating health with increasing age, index B gives evidence of a health component that improves with age. And this is despite the fact that all three health variables are strongly positively correlated.

Discussion

These analyses show that the symptom index is not an adequate measure of general health, despite the fact that standard validation procedures found no problems with the scale. The results are actually quite disturbing the moment we note the contradictory results obtained by different versions of the symptom index:

1 The original index with 12 items was not associated with age.
2 Index A consisting of 6 items was positively correlated with age.
3 Index B (the remaining 6 items) was negatively correlated with age.

There are obvious problems with objectivity here. It is possible to obtain any kind of result concerning the age–health relationship by constructing an index scale in the right (or wrong) way. And this is despite the fact that a relatively careful psychometric analysis of validity found no problems with the scale! We suggest that the many contradictory results published on the existence and nature of the relationship between age and symptom indices originate in exactly this problem.

Of special importance, we note that repeated findings that a number of symptoms and self-reported health are related – a result that also surfaced in this study – did not guarantee that the index symptom was valid and adequate. Correlation, even partial correlation, may be a necessary requirement for validity, but it is not a sufficient condition.

The same reservation may of course be expressed in connection with self-reported health scales. Correlations with symptoms do not guarantee the validity of SRH, both because correlations obviously are not enough in themselves, and also because symptom indices are not generally valid. One cannot argue for validity with reference to an invalid scale.

That this study did not find any problems with the two separate index scales does not mean that we think that health is two dimensional. The analysis raises several questions that can only be answered theoretically, even though the results of the larger study, including a larger number of items and a wider range of exogenous variables, broadly confirm what has been reported here: the major source of heterogeneity among items has to do with age more than anything else. A two-dimensional symptom index is an adequate measure of general health for this study.

Concerning procedures for validation of index scales (of any kind), these findings have several implications. The first and most important is never to rely completely on previously reported validations of a given scale. We could regard the initial psychometric validation of the symptom index as a previous validation reported elsewhere. The validation was successful in its own terms, but unfortunately missed the point of this study: whether or not the scale was adequate for analysis aimed at a specific variable of intrinsic interest. Age probably would always be one of the exogenous variables included in a validation study, but other studies might focus on exogenous variables that were not included in this investigation.

Secondly, some validation techniques do appear in several different contexts after all. Analysis of item bias and a check of the conditional Rasch model (and thereby the exchangeability of items) will appear in the same way, whether or not we include an intervening latent variable between the symptom index and the exogenous variables. The validation procedure tells us nothing at all about whether or not a latent structure model is to be preferred to a model with only manifest variables.

Finally we note that certain problems have not been dealt with at all in this chapter. Missing exogenous variables will have consequences for conditional independence of items, but not for the appearance of the conditional Rasch model. This is another indication that a check of the conditional Rasch model is at best a partial check of the properties of the scale. The problems with index scales appearing as explanatory variables in causal or recursive models are quite different from the problems with the index scales for random responses that we have dealt with in this chapter.

References

Andersen, E.B. (1977) 'Sufficient statistics and latent trait models', *Psykometrika*, 42: 69–81.

Andersen, E.B. (1980) *Discrete Statistical Models with Social Science Applications*. Amsterdam: North Holland.

Andrich, D. (1988) *Rasch Models for Measurement*. Sage University Paper Series on Quantitative Applications in the Social Sciences, 68. Beverly Hills and London: Sage.

Borhnstedt, G.W. (1983) 'Measurement', in P. Rossi, J. Wright and A. Anderson (eds), *Handbook of Survey Research*. New York: Academic Press. pp. 70–122.

Cockerham, W.C., Sharp, K. and Wilcox, J.A. (1983) 'Aging and perceived health status', *Journal of Gerontology*, 38: 349–55.

Davis, J.A. (1967) 'A partial coefficient for Goodman and Kruskal's gamma', *Journal of the American Statistical Association*, 69: 174–80.

Dawid, A.P. (1979) 'Conditional independence in statistical theory (with discussion)', *Journal of the Royal Statistical Society, Series B*. 41: 1–31.

Dean, K. (1986) 'Social support and health: pathways of influence', *Health Promotion*, 1: 133–50.

Fillenbaum, G.G. (1979) 'Social context and self-assessment of health among the elderly', *Journal of Health and Social Behavior*, 20: 45–51.

Fornell, C. and Yi, Y. (1992) 'Assumptions of the two-step approach to latent variable modeling', *Social Methods and Research*, 20: 291–320.

Gustafsson, J.-E. (1980) 'Testing and obtaining fit of data to the Rasch model', *British Journal of Mathematical and Statistical Psychology*, 33: 205–33.

Jylhä, M., Leskinen, E., Alanen, E., Leskinen, A.L. and Heikkinen, E. (1986) 'Self-rated health and associated factors among men of different ages', *Journal of Gerontology*, 41: 710–16.

Kreiner, S. (1986) *Computerized Exploratory Screening of Large Dimensional Contingency Tables*. Compstat, Proceedings in Computational Statistics. 7th Symposium Rome: 43–8. Heidelberg: Physica Verlag.

Linn, B.S. and Linn, M.W. (1980) 'Objective and self-assessed health in the old and very old', *Social Science and Medicine*, 14A: 311–15.

Lord, F.M. (1980) *Applications of Item Response Theory to Practical Testing Problems*. New Jersey: Lawrence Erlbaum.

Murray, J., Dunn, G. and Tarnopolsky, A. (1982) 'Self-assessment of health: an exploration of the effects of physical and psychological symptoms', *Psychological Medicine*, 12: 371–8.

Osterlind, S.J. (1983) *Test Item Bias*. Sage University Paper Series on Quantitative Applications in the Social Sciences, 30. Berverly Hills and London: Sage.

Rasch, G. (1960/1980) *Probabilistic Models for some Intelligence and Attainment Tests*. Copenhagen: Danish Institute for Educational Research, 1960. Expanded edition, Chicago: University of Chicago Press, 1980.

Rasch, G. (1966) 'An item analysis which takes individual differences into account', *British Journal of Mathematical and Statistical Psychology*, 19: 49–57.

Rosenbaum, P. (1989) 'Criterion-related Construct Validity', *Psychometrika*, 54: 625–34.

Thornstam, L. (1975) 'Health and self-perceptions', *The Gerontologist*, 15: 264–70.

Tjur, T. (1982) 'A connection between Rasch's item analysis model and a multiplicative Poisson model', *Scandinavian Journal of Statistics*, 9: 23–30.

Whittaker, J. (1990) *Graphical Models in Applied Multivariate Analysis*. New York: Wiley.

7

Some Aspects of Statistical Models

David Cox

Introduction

This chapter deals in broad terms with some issues connected with the analysis and interpretation of empirical data arising in health research; most of the matters occur in similar form in other contexts.

The reliable information essential for the advancement of knowledge may take a number of different forms, including:

1. Impressionistic information obtained, for example, from largely unstructured interviews with a small number of representative or key or unusually interesting individuals.
2. Data obtained by careful observation of a very small number of individuals, perhaps even a single individual.
3. Historical data compiled, possibly incidentally in some administrative process or for some other purpose, and now subjected to secondary analysis.
4. Data obtained via a planned observational or experimental study and now subjected to primary analysis. The analysis of such data in a population health context is the primary focus of the present book.

All these have a role, the first especially in giving qualitative insight and suggesting topics and hypotheses for more detailed study, and the second both for those same reasons and also for situations where individual patient management is difficult and requires frequent monitoring and possible changes of treatment regime. The recent literature on so-called $n=1$ trials has statistical aspects. We shall here, however, concentrate largely on the fourth form – primary analysis of planned studies.

Science is an essentially public activity, and science-based technology thrives on information that can be subject to public appraisal and criticism. Thus the use of clearly defined and widely understood statistical methods of various kinds plays a key role. If data of any substance are obtained, they must be summarized for interpretation in a generally understandable way, and in this some form of statistical analysis, whether it be via simple graphs and tables or by more complex techniques, is entirely unavoidable.

It is fruitless to draw a rigid distinction between the general principles of scientific investigation and statistical notions, and in some sense statistical considerations are involved in all the following phases:

(a) formulation of objectives
(b) design of study
(c) piloting of data collection
(d) data collection and monitoring of data quality
(e) preliminary analysis
(f) 'final' analysis of data
(g) formulation of conclusions
(h) subject-matter interpretation of conclusions
(i) presentation of conclusions, whether verbally or in published form, these calling for rather different approaches, implementation and/or formulation of more work.

The implications are both that some knowledge of statistical ideas (concepts rather than specific techniques) is important for all investigators, and also that some involvement of a statistician as a full member of a collaborative team, taking part in all or most discussions and familiar with the subject-matter background, is desirable from the start. Recent experience seems to suggest strongly that this is the most effective approach, at least in major studies. The *ad hoc* consulting of a statistician to sort out technical difficulties at the stage of detailed analysis may sometimes be enough, but is usually second best. That is, a statistician is more valuable as a collaborator than as a consultant.

We have already stressed that statistical methods are not confined to formal methods involving probability models, although that is the main emphasis of the present chapter. By 'model' in this chapter we always mean statistical model, although of course the word can be used much more widely to mean, in particular, the idealized framework within which a particular investigation or set of data are to be viewed. In some contexts it is important to stress that data do not stand on their own, but have always to be viewed in terms of some implicit or explicit assumptions.

Probability and Statistical Models

The notion of probability enters statistical discussions in two different although strongly related ways, corresponding to the ideas of uncertainty of knowledge and variability of observed outcome. It is a feature of statistical analysis that one recognizes conclusions to be subject to error or uncertainty and that one aims to measure this uncertainty explicitly and quantitatively; probability is a key tool in doing this. Uncertainty arises also in studying decisions made by professionals and clients in contexts with incomplete information. We shall here, however, concentrate on the second interpretation of probability as a way of representing uncontrolled variability encountered in the real world, recognizing that virtually all real investigations involve data containing such unexplained variation.

To take a specific example, it would be absurd to regard the diastolic blood pressure of Danish males as defined by a single number. Even if we are more specific and specify a male to be healthy in some defined sense, and of age 50 years, height 1.95 m and weight 75 kg, we must still think of a distribution of values and consider the probability that the diastolic blood pressure is less than 80 mm Hg, 90 mm Hg and so on. It is this distribution of probability that characterizes the situation, not a single number. In practice the situation is even more complicated because it may be crucial that there is variation not only between individuals but between times for a given individual, variation between different observers, and so on. Thus we may need to treat haphazard variation as having a complex structure. The techniques of components of variance and covariance provide powerful and somewhat underused tools for analysing haphazard variation, recognizing especially that key properties of individuals are often not stable in time. A merging of these techniques with those of time series analysis is one potentially fruitful topic for methodological development, as also are the extensions to qualitative and ordered data.

To recognize that such variability exists at all seems crucial for straight thinking. A statistical model carries this step a stage further by formulating an idealized mathematical representation of the form of the variation using the concept of a probability distribution. In the present context it might take the form that in the population under study the log of diastolic blood pressure has a special mathematical form of distribution called a normal or Gaussian distribution defined by a parameter σ, the standard deviation, which measures variability, and by a parameter μ, the mean, which itself has some such structure as

$$\nu + \beta_1 \text{ age (years)} + \beta_2 \log \text{height (m)} + \beta_3 \log \text{weight (kg)} \qquad (7.1)$$

In this the Greek letters represent population properties which are unknown parameters to be estimated from relevant data. For example, β_3 is the mean increase in log mm Hg of diastolic blood pressure per unit increase in log weight, estimated as we compare in the population the men of the same height and age but differing weight. This is essentially the proportional change in blood pressure divided by a proportional change in weight. Note that this is not necessarily at all the same as the change that would be induced were a particular man to change his weight, for example by modification of diet or exercise.

Equation (7.1) is just one of many possibilities, and the precise form of the equation may well need modification in the light of the data.

The following general features of a statistical model are important and may have far-reaching implications:

1. The parameters refer to a particular method of measurement in a particular random system or population.
2. The model is an idealization and as such tentative and to some extent at least capable of being modified or even totally rejected in the light of the data. Thus a quite different form of dependence on age or other relevant variables may be required.
3. Interpretation will be based on estimates of key parameters which often express dependence of response variables (such as blood pressure) on explanatory variables (such as age). These are properties of the population estimated from the data, with an error which is assessed by the method of analysis. It is crucial to understand the subject-matter interpretation of the parameter. It is a substantial advantage if such interpretation does not depend strongly on secondary technical statistical assumptions (for example normality) necessary to complete the specification of the model.
4. If the dependencies and interrelationships are of complex or subtle kind, it may be important that models of comparable subtlety are used. There is a difficult clash here. If there is a golden rule of statistical analysis, it is to use the simplest methods adequate for the job. With careful design it may be possible to address subtle issues by simple methods, but it is likely, especially with observational rather than experimental studies, that the methods of analysis employed need to be of a complexity matching that of the issues addressed.

There are four broad reasons for introducing relatively complex models into the analysis of data. First, in some cases, via the use of substantive models, they allow important subject-matter considerations to be taken account of. Secondly, they provide, via the notion of a parameter, a way of summarizing key aspects of the system under study via one or more interpretable numbers. Thirdly, they provide a way of assessing the uncertainty of conclusions, or at least of that part of the uncertainty that is connected with having observed only a limited amount of data (the sample) rather than the whole random system (the population). Finally, they provide, via the concepts and techniques of theoretical statistics, a way of developing methods of analysis that are in a certain sense efficient in extracting all the information in the data, subject to the broad adequacy of the model postulated as the basis of the analysis.

Classification of Models

For the present purpose it is useful to consider two main types of model, the substantive and the empirical. For a more detailed development see Cox (1990), who introduced also a third type, the so-called indirect models, which we shall not discuss here because they are not directly relevant for the primary or secondary analysis of data.

Broadly speaking the distinction is that the substantive models but not the empirical introduce specific subject-matter considerations. Thus the equation for mean log diastolic blood pressure in the previous section is not based on any special physiological theory but rather is an attempt to represent changes in diastolic blood pressure as smooth with respect to the explanatory variables in question. It is at the same time the strength and the weakness of empirical models that virtually the same formal model can usefully represent a wide range of phenomena.

Substantive models are of two broad types. The first represents, even if in very idealized form, underlying mechanisms or processes, for example pharmacological or biochemical. The second represents hypotheses generated by subject-matter considerations, the research hypotheses of Wermuth and Lauritzen (1989), expressing combinations of strong dependencies and conditional independencies. A typical example of the second is that, given some current physiological measurements on a patient, some medical outcome variable, such as survival, is independent of some variables concerning medical or social background; in a sense, the current physiological variables capture all that is relevant for the patient's survival. This is a representation of an underlying process, but only a rather qualitative representation. Note that to some extent the language of hypotheses is just a useful convention. It would amount to much the same to say that it would be of subject-matter interest to examine the direction and magnitude of the conditional relation between outcome and background variables given current physiological variables.

Of course for fuller understanding of the above situation and for matters ranging from treatment to resource allocation, considerations other than survival and certainly including health-status measures (quality of life) are essential, and more detailed study of the interrelationships among the different kinds of variable is needed. Graphical models will often be helpful for this.

Empirical models by contrast, as already stated, have no strong specific subject-matter background. Their main purpose is to summarize population relationships and distributions in a small number of parameters, some of all of which can be a basis for interpretation and which can be estimated with specified uncertainty. A second subsidiary but nevertheless important role is to serve as a basis for correcting for data deficiencies, such as incomplete observation and censoring.

In summary, substantive models represent injections of theory, quantitative or qualitative, into the analysis, whereas broadly speaking empirical models do not.

Forecasting of AIDS

As a first illustration of the issues raised above, we outline some of the considerations involved in the short-term forecasting of the AIDS epidemic in the UK. For a review of epidemiological and statistical work on this see the collection of papers edited by Anderson, Cox and Hillier (1989) and for more qualitative discussion see Report of a Working Group (1988). The primary data are the numbers of cases reported month by month together with dates of diagnosis. There is much background information.

We assume some familiarity with the main features of the epidemic, in particular that being infective as such is asymptomatic, that infection can be detected by seropositivity on test, and that there is a long and very variable incubation period between infection and the onset of AIDS.

For simplicity we ignore the issue of under-reporting and do not distinguish between cases in the different main risk groups – male homosexuals, IDUs etc. If we plot the data as number of cases per month versus month of diagnosis using data up to say 1 January 1990, we obtain a curve first rising roughly exponentially and then coming to a maximum in mid to late 1989 before dropping away. This decrease is an artefact of reporting delays, which range from a few weeks to one or two years. Many of the cases diagnosed in late 1989 are 'missing' but will become available in due course. It is a typical illustration of the second type of empirical model to adjust for this. If $\rho_d(t)$ is the rate of diagnosis at time t, the observed rate of diagnosis at time t, $\rho_{od}(t)$ say, is given by

$$\rho_{od}(t) = \int_{-\infty}^{t_0} F_X\,(t_0-u)\,\rho_d(u)\mathrm{d}u$$

where $F_X\,(t-t_0)$ is the probability that a reporting lag X is less than t_0-t where t_0 is the time at which the data collection is closed, that is 1 January 1990 in our example. We have no substantive theory to guide us as to the choice of $F_X(x)$ and so we make an empirical fitting of a flexible functional form of distribution, not a totally straightforward matter, and in effect use the estimated F to adjust the observed $\rho_{od}(t)$ to the required $\rho_d(t)$.

A major conceptual issue arises over the nature of probability in a context like this. The data show substantial erratic fluctuations as well as trend, and the function $\rho_d(t)$ is considered to be a smooth function representing a 'true' or population rate. Stochastic fluctuations around this are represented by a special process called a time-dependent Poisson process. This probability model accounts both for trend and, although imperfectly, for the fluctuations around the trend. The supposition is that, at least for some purposes, the full UK data are a sample from a hypothetical population of values that would be generated if the same underlying process operated on a very large scale.

For prediction we have in effect to estimate the rate of diagnosis $\rho_d(t)$ from the data and then extrapolate the function to the time range of interest. There are essentially four ways of doing this, all involving some kind of statistical modelling. These methods are briefly as follows.

The first method is to assume that the epidemic in the UK will approximately follow the course in the US but with a time lag. That is, we assume that approximately

$$\rho_d^{UK}\,(t) = \alpha\,\rho_d^{US}\,(t-\gamma)$$

where α is a ratio of effective population sizes and γ is a time lag. Roughly γ=2.5 years so that, good data being available from the US, forecasting for at least that period is possible, once the rate for the US has been reasonably estimated. Among the limitations of this approach are effects of improved treatment procedures invalidating the key comparison, and the fact that the balance of risk groups is not the same in the two countries.

The second method goes back to first principles but is difficult to apply to the AIDS epidemic. This is first to estimate the process of infection, to regard as known the distribution of incubation time and the proportion who will convert to AIDS, and then to use a mathematical relation between rate of infection, rate of diagnosis at a subsequent time and the distribution of incubation time to predict $\rho_d(t)$. This approach can be followed to a limited extent but only indirectly, because for AIDS infection is not observable and little is known about the rate of new infections. See, however, Isham (1989) and Day et al. (1989) for an ingenious back projection method.

The third method is to construct a moderately realistic mathematical model of the progression of the epidemic (Anderson et al., 1989). The resulting differential equations can be solved numerically and in principle projected into the future for as long as required. This approach, which is a strong form of substantive model, is of great interest for gaining understanding of the primary determining features of the epidemic, but the snag for short-term quantitative forecasting is that large numbers of parameters have to be estimated or assigned values in the light of general knowledge of the epidemic. To be at all realistic such a model, even if confined to male homosexuals, has to take account of heterogeneous levels of sexual behaviour (for example rate of partner change), changes in sexual practices with time, variable incubation periods, probable changes in infectivity as the incubation period develops, and so on. Methods for the systematic fitting of models of this level of complexity are not available.

The fourth method, the most straightforward, is to assume a suitable mathematical form for the rate of diagnosis $\rho_d(t)$, to estimate it from the incidence data, allowing for reporting delays as indicated above, and then to extrapolate. The difficulty here is the choice of mathematical form, since goodness of fit is determined by the behaviour in the range of the data, and functions very similar over the data may extrapolate quite differently. This is an argument against empirical modelling, that is the choice of $\rho_d(t)$ without regard to subject-matter considerations. A reasonable approach, which is that of going some of the way towards a substantive model, is to be guided in model choice by the conclusions from the strongly substantive models, discussed briefly in the previous method. Most theoretical models show an initial phase of exponential growth followed by transition to a regime of much slower growth, not far from linear; eventually a maximum is reached. This suggests, in the present context, fitting a function which starts exponentially and then switches to approximate linearity. Such a form is the linear logistic, namely

$$\rho_d(t) = (\rho_1 + \rho_2 t)\{1 + \rho_1\rho_3 \exp(-\rho_4 t)\}^{-1}$$

There remain substantial technical problems of fitting and uncertainty assessment, but this seems a reasonably sensible approach, at least for the UK.

The arguments sketched above illustrate some of the combinations of empirical and substantive modelling often needed in relatively complicated applications. Note that the second and third are at least in part substantive models, whereas the fourth is an empirical model whose broad form is suggested by theoretical considerations; there is no rigid distinction between the two types of model!

Measurement of Quality of Life

As a quite different example we consider some aspects of a large subject, the measurement of health status, or what is sometimes rather grandiosely called quality of life. This arises in at least three contexts, of which we consider mainly the first:

1 comparison of treatments in clinical trials in which survival, blood pressure control or other 'objectively' measured responses are not the primary or at least not the sole basis of comparison, but self-assessed well-being or absence of side effects are important
2 the choice by individual patients between alternative regimes with different risky consequences
3 the study of health resource allocation on the basis of maximizing some measure of gain achieved.

There is a rapidly growing literature on these topics. For an early but still valuable review see Fayers and Jones (1983), and for a more detailed discussion, but still concentrating on clinical trials, see Cox et al. (1992).

In some cases simple measures are adequate, such as: working, yes or no; in hospital, yes or no; walking, yes or no. In most cases, however, a battery of questions concerning relevant aspects of physical, mental and social activity are considered as well as questions on the absence or, if present, the severity of various side effects. There are a large number of statistical aspects concerned with the design of studies, the design of instruments, the testing of instruments and the analysis of data. On the whole, in the absence of strong underlying quantitative theory, models tend to be empirical.

Suppose, however, that we have data on physical and biochemical features that are not directly symptomatic, 'objective' measures of health status, such as the results of exercise tests, and self-assessed measures of well-being. Then a substantive hypothesis might be that treatments affect physical and biochemical variables, which in turn determine 'objective' status, which in turn determines self-assessed status. This amounts to a substantive hypothesis of some strong dependencies plus conditional independence between various sets of variables:

(a) Objective status is conditionally independent of treatment given physical variables.
(b) Self-assessed status is conditionally independent of treatment and physical variables given objective status.

The 'theory' expressed in these hypotheses is no doubt simplistic in the extreme but all the same could be a useful starting point for interpretation, for example via graphical chain models.

For the analysis of self-assessed questionnaire data one possible approach, which goes some way towards a substantive model, postulates underlying observed (latent) 'true' measures of physical etc. well-being from which the observations deviate by random amounts. This leads to so-called psychometric methods in which relatively complicated calculations lead to scores to be attached to the different answers to each question. While in general substantive models are probably to be preferred to empirical models it seems likely that in the present applications, although perhaps not in instrument development, it is better to use simpler methods leading to simpler analysis via unweighted means of simple scores. Here empirical models are natural in which, after representing subject, time and treatment effects, all responses of a particular type have the same variance and all pairs are equally correlated. Observations of two different types on an individual can also be assumed to have equal but lower correlation. This is a convenient framework for a simple analysis in terms of category totals and for the assessment of anomalous individuals, questions or categories.

For detailed analysis, interpretation and understanding it is necessary to keep the distinct dimensions of quality of life separate. Not only is a system of weighting used to combine them into a single measure likely to be arbitrary but, more fundamentally, the relative importance attached to the different dimensions varies greatly between individuals; it is very desirable to recognize such variations in, for example, assessing health care measures (Cox et al., 1992).

Generalizability of Conclusions

There are many general issues implicitly raised by the present topic. We shall consider only one: that of the generality of the conclusions from a particular investigation.

It is almost a necessary condition for an effect to be of scientific rather than anecdotal interest that it can, under appropriate conditions, be reproduced by other investigators. In health terms a conclusion highly specific to a particular population may be of considerable local interest but is almost bound to raise the question as to whether the same conclusion holds elsewhere. The role of statistical methods in establishing the generality of conclusions is thus important. We discuss this briefly under four broad headings.

Even for the issue of forecasting AIDS in a specific country the generality of the conclusions, while superficially unimportant, should be of concern. To the extent that the pattern is not the same in different countries, such differences should be capable of epidemiological explanation and such explanation adds to understanding and hence to future predictability. In a large multicentre or multinational investigation the issue of breadth of application will to some extent be taken care of. Even in smaller studies, standard design considerations will put some emphasis on the range of validity of conclusions.

Parameters in a statistical model refer to a population of individuals, and the uncertainties involved in passing from sample to population are precisely those assessed in statistical analysis. While this gives substantial protection against overinterpretation, it is not, except in the case of sample surveys from a well-defined target population, a basis for striking generalization.

Demonstration of an absence of serious interaction of, say, a treatment effect with relevant explanatory variables, that is that the treatment effect is essentially the same whatever the values of the explanatory variables characterizing the individuals involved, does give reassurance for the stability of the effect under study. Thus if in a particular study or set of studies a treatment effect is essentially the same for men and women, for young and old, for smokers and non-smokers etc., confidence in extrapolation to a new population is considerably enhanced.

Finally, most importantly and related to the previous point, assessment of independent studies bearing on the same issue may show consistent effects. The statistical aspects of the combination of the results of independence studies have a long history. Recent emphasis on it is very welcome, although the coining of special names, meta-analysis for example, seems unnecessary; no new principles are involved. The key issues concern whether the data to be merged are mutually consistent, at least qualitatively; how to resolve or explain any inconsistencies that may be present; and, if consistency is achieved, how best to provide an overall summary and to assess its precision. Note particularly that in observational studies in which there are strong associations between explanatory variables, essentially arbitrary selections of subsets of explanatory variables as a basis for interpretation may make sensible comparisons of different studies very difficult. Important analyses of this kind have been given recently for beta-blockers, for platelet therapy and for the treatment of breast cancer.

The most powerful base for generalization is, however, understanding in some deep sense. The strategy that seems to have been most effective in the physical sciences is to achieve this via intensive study of situations in which the effects under investigation arise in their 'purest' form. It is, of course, hard to apply this approach to the very complex problems of population health research.

Role of Multivariate Methods

Most investigations of any complexity involve various types of observation on each individual. These can be classified in a number of ways, the classification depending at least to some extent on the conceptual framework in terms of which the data are to be interpreted. The main categories are:

1 Response variables, for example survival or quality of life, whose dependence on other explanatory variables is to be studied.
2 Intermediate response variables, which at some stage of analysis are responses and at another stage are explanatory. Examples, depending on context, include blood pressure and biochemical measurements on patients, which may be responses to treatment yet explanatory of survival or quality of life.
3 Explanatory variables that are treatments or quasi-treatments, that is which could conceivably be different for an individual from what is observed. Diet would sometimes, but not always, be a quasi-treatment.
4 Intrinsic variables which are conceptually fixed for an individual. Gender (for most purposes) is an example, so is date of birth, and so sometimes would be diet.
5 Non-specific variables, such as blocks, centres and clinics, corresponding to divisions of the data into sets that are likely to be different, often in many not clearly identified ways.

Recognition of these distinctions, or something closely akin to them, seems essential for careful interpretation. In experimental studies, treatment and some other variables may be controlled by the investigator; in observational studies, most variables will in a sense be random although conditioning on the observed values of the explanatory variables will usually be appropriate. Multivariate analysis in the narrow technical statistical sense involves the consideration of several response variables simultaneously. A probably quite widely held view among statisticians is that multivariate analysis is to be avoided if possible, except for empirical dimension reduction. Interrelated series of univariate analyses will indeed often be adequate and some graphical chain analyses can be viewed in this light; that is the separate pieces of the analysis may be univariate logistic or other regression analyses. The important role of the graphical chain model is to synthesize the fragments of analysis into a coherent scheme. They can be viewed as an alternative to the linear structural equation models introduced by econometricians following the remarks of Haavelmo (1943).

Situations where multivariate methods are virtually inevitable include:

(a) Those where latent variables are introduced with the objective of explaining several somewhat distinct response variables, as in linear structural relation models for continuous variables.
(b) Those where explanatory variables change the pattern of association of distinct response variables.
(c) Those cases where simultaneous response models not of recursive form are found empirically to give a particularly concise representation of complex data.

There are very different issues of strategy here which only substantial empirical experience of particular subject-matter fields can resolve.

Relation between Statistical Innovation and Substantive Research

Many scientific advances stem from developments in technique; think, for example, of the impact of modern electron microscopy and of the various forms of chromatography. It is entirely proper and fruitful that those responsible for technical developments should aim to ensure wide applicability of their ideas, in due course via relatively routinely available apparatus. Much the same is true for developments in statistical methodology, with suitable software playing the part of routine apparatus. Yet where a statistician, or group of statisticians, has developed new techniques or new software and is deeply involved in a specific application, there is a dilemma. On the one hand, there is the natural desire to see the results of applying the new methods; on the other, there is a clear imperative to use methods that are simple and are most appropriate for the substantive issues.

It is undeniably good that most theoretical statistical research workers are involved in applied statistical work. The point is that there may have to be some conscious distancing between the two lines of activity. This appears broadly; developments in survival analysis, graphical chain methods and linear structural relations are obvious examples.

Conclusion

This chapter has addressed in rather general terms a few of the strategic problems associated with the careful analysis of empirical data, and has given a slightly more detailed discussion of two specific problems. Many important matters have not been discussed, including for example procedures for model choice, the role of significance tests and the special features of work on statistical decision analysis.

There is a bewildering variety of detailed models for special purposes. While the choice of models and procedures is to some extent dictated by the availability of software, in principle the most desirable general approach for the analysis of major investigations is the use of models in line with and suggested by substantive ideas. Thereby the destructive notion of a clash between subject-matter and statistical considerations is avoided.

Note

I am very grateful to Kathryn Dean, Svend Kreiner and Nanny Wermuth for constructive comments.

References

Anderson, R.M., Blythe, S.P., Gupta, S. and Konigs, E. (1989) 'The transmission dynamics of the human immunodeficiency virus type 1 in the male homosexual community in the United Kingdom: the influence of changes in sexual behaviour', *Philosophical Transactions of the Royal Society of London, Series B*, 325: 45–98.

Anderson, R.M., Cox, D.R. and Hillier, H.C. (eds) (1989) 'Epidemiological and statistical aspects of the AIDS epidemic', *Philosophical Transactions of the Royal Society of London, Series B*, 325: 37–187.

Cox, D.R. (1990) 'The role of models in statistical analysis', *Statistical Science*, 5: 169–74.

Cox, D.R., Fitzpatrick, R., Fletcher, A., Gore, S.M., Jones, D.R. and Spiegelhalter, D. (1992) 'Quality of life assessment: can we keep it simple? (with discussion)', *Journal of the Royal Statistical Society, Series A*, 155: 353–93.

Day, N., Gore, S.M., McGee, M.A. and Smith, M. (1989) 'Predictions of the AIDS epidemic in the U.K.: the use of the back projection methods', *Philosophical Transactions of the Royal Society of London, Series B*, 325: 123–34.

Fayers, P.M. and Jones, D.R. (1983) 'Measuring and analysing quality of life data in cancer clinical trials', *Statistics in Medicine*, 2: 429–46.

Haavelmo, T. (1943) 'The statistical implications of a system of simultaneous equations, *Econometrica*, 11: 1–13.

Isham, V. (1989) 'Estimation of the incidence of HIV infection', *Philosophical Transactions of the Royal Society of London, Series B*, 325: 113–21.

Report of a Working Group, Department of Health and The Welsh Office (1988) *Short-Term Prediction of HIV Infection and AIDS in England and Wales*. London: HMSO.

Wermuth, N. and Lauritzen, S.L. (1989) 'On substantive research hypotheses, conditional independence graphs and graphical chain models (with discussion), *Journal of the Royal Statistical Society, Series B*, 52: 21–72.

8

Graphical Interaction Models: a New Approach for Statistical Modelling

Joe Whittaker

Introduction

This chapter could begin with a formal definition of the probabilistic concept of conditional independence together with a short account of its historical genesis, followed by an application to data analysis to establish its credentials as a useful tool. However, this rather dry approach may easily deter the reader with a limited mathematical background. In the hope of raising the motivation of the research worker we stress the application first, and show in the second section how a six-way contingency table may be speedily reduced to more manageable proportions. Conditional independence and its foundation role in the definition of graphical interaction models are explained in the third section, which may in some sense be simply paraphrased: the right way to examine the potentially complex pattern of interaction within a set of variables is to determine the conditions under which variables become irrelevant to other relationships. The extension to more complicated studies involving mixed discrete and continuous variables and involving hierarchies of response and explanatory variables is briefly discussed at the end of the third section. In the fourth section some of the more practical issues are addressed, such as how to use these models with relatively few observations, the problems of graphical model selection and the differences between exploratory and confirmatory analyses. Finally, in the fifth section the relationship between the diagrams used in latent variable modelling and the conditional independence graphs of graphical modelling are contrasted.

An aim of this chapter is to introduce the idea of graphical models in order to make sense of possible patterns of multivariate interaction between several measured variables. A more formal view of the graph and its construction from the perspective of probability theory shows how graphs can portray multivariate interaction, response-explanatory models such as regression, and further generalizations such as causal modelling.

Randomized Studies

To illustrate the power and wide-ranging applications of conditional independence, take for instance the question that cholesterol carries a higher risk of coronary heart disease – a matter which in principle is easy to resolve. One divides a group of representative individuals into two subgroups, one insists that one subgroup undertakes a high-cholesterol regime and the other a low-cholesterol regime for a predetermined period of years, and then, after holding all other potentially confounding variables constant (*ceteris paribus*) or at the very least at comparable levels in the two subgroups, one examines the difference in prevalence of heart disease at the end of the experiment. A difference in prevalence indicates that cholesterol is a cause of heart disease, and this may be represented by

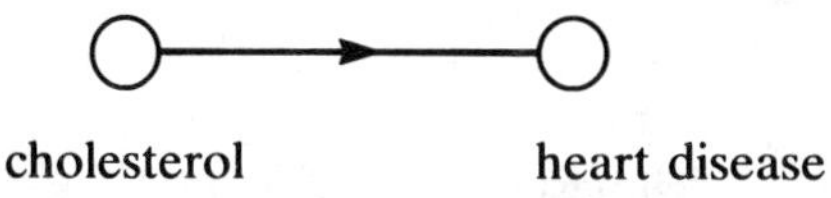

(Un?)fortunately health science does not quite work like this. The investigator, who is rarely in a position to experiment, has to resort to other, less rigorous methods. A key problem is that if individuals themselves choose their diet then any observed difference in heart disease prevalence could be argued to be due to unmeasured differences in other factors, which also have contributed to the individuals' dietary decisions. This may be portrayed diagrammatically by the graph

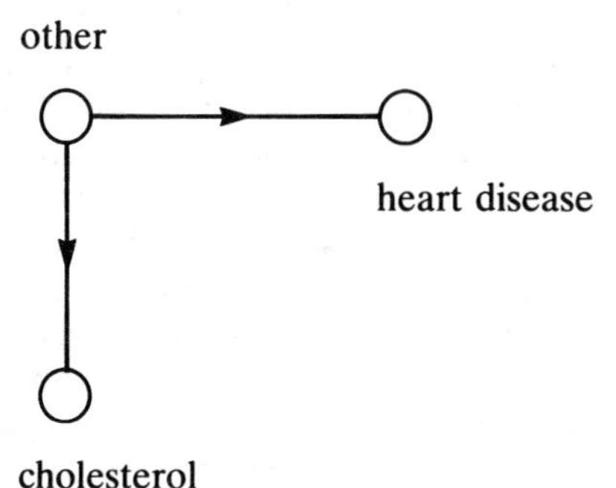

which 'explains' the observed interaction

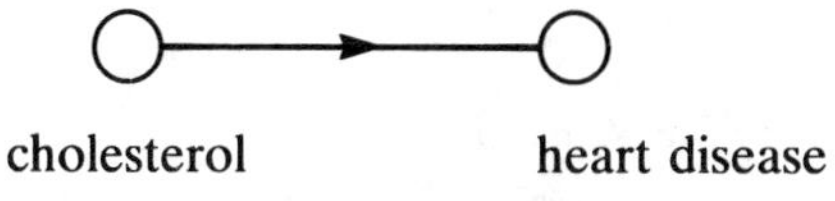

between cholesterol and coronary heart disease.

However, if it is known *a priori* that there is no possibility of interaction between other factors and cholesterol, then in the graph with three nodes there is no edge between these two vertices. In this case there is no mechanism by which an observed cholesterol–disease interaction can be explained away. It is impossible (within the theory of graphical models) to derive the graph exhibiting an interaction between cholesterol and heart disease from the graph

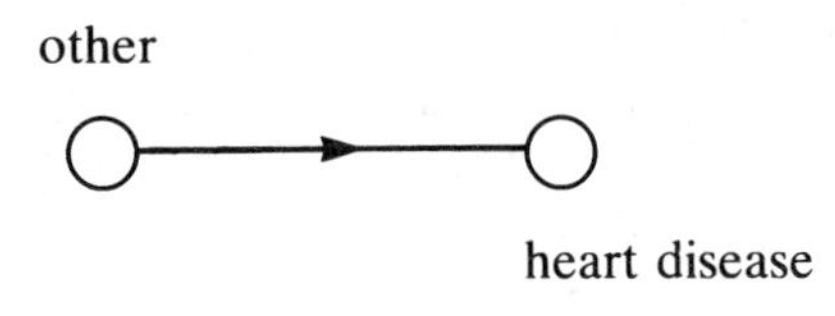

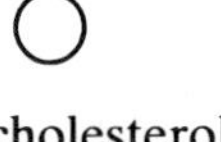

The mechanism which breaks the interaction between cholesterol uptake and other factors is randomization: the individuals in the study are assigned at random to the two regimes.

In the absence of randomized assignation, health investigators conduct an observational study and attempt to measure as many of the potential confounding factors, for example age, sex and weight, as possible. Then, if necessary, the measured association between heart disease and cholesterol is adjusted for differences in these factors, and a good deal of statistics in the health sciences involves the analysis of multivariate measures, taken on many individuals and often at many times. Analysing such information is the rationale for graphical modelling. In fact some might argue that because randomization eliminates the effect of other influences, the randomized experiment is not the most relevant context in which to investigate questions concerning population health. It is the strength of graphical modelling that its theory not only illustrates the methodology of randomization but, irrespective of its application, addresses the key question of how interaction between variables, say a potential cause and a potential effect, alters in the presence of other mediating influences.

A Case Study of Car Workers

Interaction and Balance

The information in Table 8.1 was collected at the beginning of a 15-year follow-up study of probable risk factors for coronary thrombo-

Table 8.1 *Prognostic factors in coronary heart disease*

				B:	no		yes	
F	*E*	*D*	*C*	*A*:	no	yes	no	yes
neg.	<3	<140	no		44	40	112	67
			yes		129	145	12	23
		>140	no		35	12	80	33
			yes		109	67	7	9
	>3	<140	no		23	32	70	66
			yes		50	80	7	13
		>140	no		24	25	73	57
			yes		51	63	7	16
pos.	<3	<140	no		5	7	21	9
			yes		9	17	1	4
		>140	no		4	3	11	8
			yes		14	17	5	2
	>3	<140	no		7	3	14	14
			yes		9	16	2	3
		>140	no		4	0	13	11
			yes		5	14	4	4

Source: Whittaker, 1990

sis, comprising data on all 1841 men employed in a Czechoslovakian car factory. The six variables that cross-classify the table are all binary and denote the following:

A smoking: no, yes
B strenuous mental work: no, yes
C strenuous physical work: no, yes
D systolic blood pressure: <140, >140
E ratio of beta and alpha lipoproteins: <3, >3
F family anamnesis of coronary heart disease: negative, positive.

There is no reason to suppose that these six possible risk factors have a treatment–response structure, and we shall treat them all on an equal footing.

Even the most cursory glance over the table reveals that each category of worker is not equally represented in this class-classification. What does this mean? First, it indicates that some variables may be associated: for example, there may be a higher frequency of high-blood-pressure subjects within the smokers than within the non-smokers. It is then natural to ask which variables are associated with which, and to what degree.

Secondly, in the context of the prospective nature of this study, where a central aim is to evaluate the risk factors for coronary heart

Table 8.2 *A fictitious two-way table*

	$Y = 1$	$Y = 2$	Total
$X = 1$	10	20	30
$X = 2$	30	60	90
Total	40	80	120

Table 8.3 *An unbalanced fictitious two-way table*

	$Y = 1$	$Y = 2$	Total
$X = 1$	50	10	60
$X = 2$	10	50	60
Total	60	60	120

disease, that the cell entries differ means there is a lack of balance in the study. That is to say, in the follow-up phase, heart disease rates for different categories of workers will not be equally well estimated. The balanced study is desirable in that it allows separate estimates of the factors' effects on heart disease. However, in the population context, where several variables may mutually affect each other, the advantage of a study reflecting the existing uneven distribution of subjects is that the overall magnitude of heart disease can be assessed.

It is our contention that a graphical interaction model is an excellent vehicle to characterize and summarize the interaction between the measured variables and to quantify the lack of balance in the prospective study.

First note that, since the comparison of rates is of prime interest, it is not so much unequal numbers as unequal proportions that constitute imbalance or interaction. For example, in Table 8.2 the relative preponderance of $Y = 2$ observations over $Y = 1$ observations is a ratio of 2:1 irrespective of whether X is 1 or 2 or is unspecified as in the total category. The table is balanced, and the comparison of heart disease rates in the categories $Y = 2$ and $Y = 1$ does not depend on the value of X. Similarly the preponderance of $X = 2$ over $X = 1$ is 3:1 for all categories of Y.

On the other hand, in Table 8.3 most of the information is concentrated in the categories ($X = 1, Y = 1$) and ($X = 2, Y = 2$). If there is a difference in the heart disease rates here it is impossible to assign this unequivocally to the effect of X or to the effect of Y. In extremes this may vitiate the whole purpose of the survey.

Note that if the counts in these two tables are replaced by proportions then Table 8.2 exhibits independence because, for instance, $10/120 = (30/120)(40/120)$ according to the multiplication law of probabilities, and we write $X \perp\!\!\!\perp Y$. This may be portrayed by the independence graph

(X)   (Y)

which has two vertices and no edge between them. However, Table 8.3 does not because $50/120 \neq (60/120)(60/120)$ and so is represented by

(X)——(Y)

In statistical terms, balance has the consequence that the effects of different variables on heart disease are (approximately) additive and uncorrelated, a fact which dramatically simplifies the problem of statistical inference. In a prospective survey, to best evaluate the individual effects of each risk factor on coronary heart disease, it is preferable to have a completely balanced design; and if it were possible to assign individuals to groups this design would be chosen. Failing this we should at least determine and quantify the lack of balance due to interacting variables, or equivalently, the magnitude and direction of departures from the complete mutual independence of all the variables.

Finally, while this investigation is motivated by considerations of balance, it is also perfectly justifiable to simply wonder how these potential explanatory variables interact together.

A Two-Way Marginal Approach

It is not easy to determine by casual inspection if a table is balanced, as can be ascertained by glancing at Table 8.1. A straightforward method might be to examine marginal tables obtained by summing Table 8.1 over certain categories. For example, consider the two-way Table 8.4 classified by the first two variables, smoking A and mental work B. The fitted values under independence $A \perp\!\!\!\perp B$ are

Table 8.4 *A two-way marginal table and fitted values*

	A = no		A = yes		Total
B = no	522	(554.9)	541	(508.1)	1063
B = yes	439	(406.1)	339	(371.9)	778
Total	961		880		1841

given in parentheses. For instance in the category (A = no, B = no) the fitted value is 1841(1063/1841)(961/1841) = 554.9. Note that the total of the fitted values agrees with the total of the observed values.

A standard test for independence is Pearson's chi-squared statistic

$$\sum_{\text{cells}} (\text{observed} - \text{fitted})^2 / \text{fitted} = 9.648$$

which is to be compared against the tables of the chi-square distribution on 1 d.f. An alternative is the log-likelihood-ratio test statistic, also called the deviance, and defined by

$$2 \sum_{\text{cells}} \text{observed} \times \log (\text{observed} / \text{fitted}) = 9.664$$

These statistics are virtually identical in all but rather small samples; we shall prefer the latter, and we write is as dev ($A \perp\!\!\!\perp B$). If the null hypothesis of independence is true, this statistic also has (in large samples) a chi-squared distribution with one degree of freedom, and a significance test consists of comparing the observed test statistic with the critical value from the tables.

On this two-way table classifying smoking and strenuous mental work, the observed p-value is 0.0019. Clearly one would reject the hypothesis of independence and conclude that the observed association cannot be attributed to chance fluctuations.

A Three-Way Approach

The difficulty with this marginal analysis is that the observed $A \times B$ association could perhaps be explained by the separate interaction of both variables with a third variable. Consider breaking the two-way Table 8.4 down by strenuous physical work C, and forming the two two-way tables classifying A and B by C = yes and by C = no as in Table 8.5. In the first slice with C = no the deviance against independence is 2.1995. We may write

$$\text{dev}\ (A \perp\!\!\!\perp B \mid \text{C} = \text{no}) = 2.1995$$

and find the p-value is 0.1381. In the second,

$$\text{dev}\ (A \perp\!\!\!\perp B \mid C = \text{yes}) = 3.7882$$

with a p-value of 0.0516. The combined test that A and B are independent at both levels of C is

$$\text{dev}\ (A \perp\!\!\!\perp B \mid C) = 2.1995 + 3.7882 = 5.9876$$

on 2 d.f. The p-value associated with this combined test is 0.0501 and does not reach the 5 per cent level. Thus we have established that A and B are independent in the two slices of the three-way

Table 8.5 *The two-way table classified by a third variable*

	B = no		B = yes	
	A = no	A = yes	A = no	A = yes
C = no	146	122	394	265
C = yes	376	419	45	74

table corresponding to C = no and C = yes, while they are not independent in the $A \times B$ margin. Here we have an instance of the well-known phenomenon that the observed marginal pairwise interaction is explained by the interaction with a third variable; in consequence we may draw the conclusion that to rely on an analysis confined to inspection of the two-way marginal tables can lead to misleading results.

Graphical Representation

A useful way to represent these findings is by means of (conditional independence) graphs. The analysis of the two-way Table 8.4 is summarized by

The analysis of the three-way Table 8.5 is summarized by

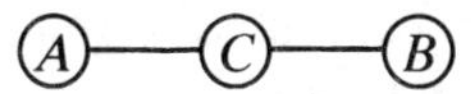

in which there is no direct connection between A and B. The relationship that A and B are independent given C is mapped into a graph in which C separates A and B. Furthermore the graph with three vertices suggests that if C were not observed then an observed interaction might be induced between A and B as each are connected to C. We shall return to this 'elastic band effect' later.

A k-Way Approach

The idea of adjusting a pair of variables for possible interaction with a third variable can be extended to an arbitrary set of variables. Suppose the variables are labelled $A_1, A_2, \ldots, A_k$. Consider a test for $A_1 \perp\!\!\!\perp A_2$ adjusting for $A_3, \ldots, A_k$. If each of the variables is binary there are 2^{k-2} $A_I \times A_2$ tables or slices. The combined test for pairwise independence modified to allow for potential interaction with all the other variables is the sum of the individual deviances from each of these 2^{k-2} slices of the full table. This adjusted test statistic is called an edge exclusion deviance.

The full set of $\binom{k}{2}$ edge exclusion deviances is a better indicator of the pattern of interaction than the $\binom{k}{2}$ tests in all the marginal tables

Table 8.6 *Edge exclusion deviances for the car worker data*

A	*					
B	22.65	*				
C	42.80	684.99	*			
D	28.72	12.23	14.81	*		
E	40.02	17.24	18.63	31.06	*	
F	21.31	22.79	22.15	18.35	18.32	*
	A	*B*	*C*	*D*	*E*	*F*

because each allows for a potential explanation in terms of the other variables. To begin, the $\binom{6}{2} = 15$ edge exclusion deviances are computed as in Table 8.6. Each entry is a test for independence at each of the $2^{6-2} = 16$ levels of the four remaining variables. Hence there are 16 d.f. associated with each chi-squared distribution, so that the critical value for a test at the 5 per cent significance level is 26.30.

The information in the edge exclusion deviance matrix is immediately revealing when combined into a single picture to give the conditional independence graph of the $k = 6$ variables. The graph is defined by the fact that pairs of variables that are not directly connected are conditionally independent given the remaining variables. Excluding the edges with non-significant deviances gives the independence graph of Figure 8.1.

Conclusions for the Car Worker Data

Figure 8.1 summarizes the pattern of interaction among the six risk factors. The complete independence of family history of *F* from the other variables is a surprise, as coronary heart disease and systolic blood pressure are both thought to be partially hereditary. Otherwise the graph suggests a coherent ordering for the variables: history–behaviour–biology.

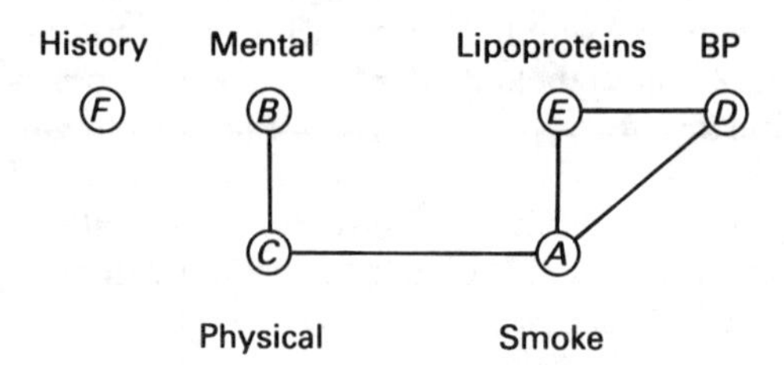

Figure 8.1 *The conditional independence graph for the car worker data*

The fact that the vertex F is not connected to the other vertices (complete independence) means that the pattern of variation between the other five variables is the same for those subjects with a family history of heart disease and for those without. Hence a single description of the five-variable pattern is available by collapsing (summing) the six-way table over the two levels of family history.

The graph shows that the six-way table can be collapsed *without* loss of information into the marginal tables classified by F, by $B \times C$, by $A \times C$ and by $A \times E \times D$; so further analysis of the interaction can continue in the one one-way, two two-way and one three-way tables. This substantially reduces the dimension of the original table while retaining all the important associations.

The graph shows that the interaction between A and B in the two-way Table 8.2 can be explained by C but now in the wider context of six interacting variables. Furthermore, one could also predict that the interaction (if any) between E and C in their two-way table could be explained by A. Marginalizing the six-way table over A may induce interaction between (E, D) and C.

It is apparent that the $B \times C$ margin needs detailed inspection. The large exclusion deviance is due to the approximate dichotomous nature of the variables. Presumably strenuous mental and physical work are approximate surrogates for blue and white collar workers in the factory.

Apart from $B \times C$ interaction, the magnitude of these dependencies is small. When divided by the sample size, each deviance is an estimate of the amount of information against the corresponding independence hypothesis, and, as $N = 1841$, these values are very small. In this sense the paradigm of complete balance is not exactly attained, but with the exception of the $B \times C$ interaction it is very nearly so.

Theory and Extensions

We make no attempt to give a historical overview of graphical modelling, but would like to point out that the essential ideas come from the pioneering work of the geneticist Sewell Wright who developed the technique of path analysis back in the 1920s (Wright, 1921; 1923). The modern mathematical theory stems from the seminal paper of Darroch et al. (1980). There are two components to the mathematical theory underpinning this technique. One is probabilistic, rooted in the notion of conditional independence, and leads to the correspondence between the separation properties of the graph and the independence statements. The other is statistical and is based on parameterizing a family of statistical distributions, such as the multivariate normal distribution, so that setting certain parameters to zero eliminates edges from the graph. A full but fairly elementary discussion is given in Whittaker (1990), which we attempt to summarize briefly here.

Conditional Independence

Conditional independence is defined as follows: A, B and C are random variables that take values in finite sets and correspond to the variables classifying the table; A is independent of B given C is written as $A \perp\!\!\!\perp B \mid C$ and is true if and only if

$$P(A \cap B \mid C) = P(A \mid C)P(B \mid C)$$

for all values of A and B and for all values of C for which $P(C) > 0$. (In fact it will be assumed that the probabilities for all cells in the table are non-zero.) An excellent review is given by Dawid (1979).

The vertices of the graph represent the random variables under consideration, and the edges of the graph embody the relationship of conditional independence. In the graph with three vertices $\{A, B, C\}$ the edge between A and B is missing if and only if $A \perp\!\!\!\perp B \mid C$:

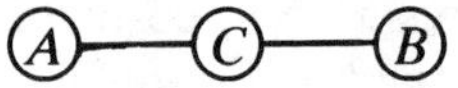

(A)—(C)—(B)

The notion is extended to $A \perp\!\!\!\perp B \mid (C, D, \ldots, K)$ when the joint distribution of several variables is considered, and for brevity this is written as $A \perp\!\!\!\perp B \mid rest$, where the *rest* designates all other variables in the set. Thus the defining relationship of the independence graph is that of pairwise independence conditioned on the remaining variables.

The resulting independence graph has certain important theoretical properties. It is Markov in the sense that (1) any pair of non-adjacent variables is independent given only the values of those variables that separate the pair; and (2) there is no better predictor for one variable from the others than those that are nearest neighbours in the graph. In consequence the graph succinctly represents the pattern of multivariate interaction.

The theory also makes important predictions about what happens when one variable (or more) is not observed, and is marginalized out from the joint distribution. One in particular can be called the *elastic band marginalization effect*, which gets its name by supposing that the edges are made of elastic and the vertices are thumbtacks, and the effect of removing a thumbtack is for the elastic to spring back to its minimal energy configuration. For example, marginalizing over variable B (removing the thumbtack at B) in the graph

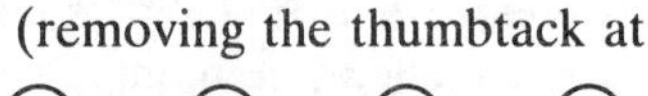

(A)—(B)—(C)—(D)

induces an edge between A and C but not between A and D. It is easy to construct examples of distributions which show this effect.

Graphical Interaction Models

Statistics enters the picture because of the need to operationalize the notion of conditional independence when dealing with data. The idea is to model the observed data as a realization from a probability experiment whose probability mechanism embodies the independence constraints inherent in the given graph. More formally, a graphical model is a family of distributions for the observed data that is indexed by free parameters which are constrained by the graph. The practical consequence is that the distribution of test statistics can be calculated which provide the tools to compare and select models to represent the data.

The binomial distribution gives the probability that a given number of heads and tails occur in n independent throws of a biased coin with probabilities p and $1 - p$. For a contingency table such as the car worker data in Table 8.1, the appropriate family of distributions is the cross-classified multinomial distribution, a generalization of the binomial distribution to several rather than just two categories. To fit a graphical model means insisting that the probabilities of the categories satisfy the conditional independence statements in the graph but are otherwise arbitrary. For example, the multinomial distribution appropriate to Table 8.4 has parameters p_{11}, p_{12}, p_{21} and p_{22}, where p_{11} is the true probability that a car worker does not smoke A and does not engage in strenuous mental activity B. If $A \perp\!\!\!\perp B$ then $p_{11} = p_{1+}\, p_{+1}$, by the multiplication rule of probability. Here $p_{1+} = p_{11} + p_{12}$. Hence the value of p_{11} is constrained by the independence graph

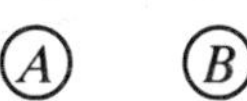

but its value is not determined as p_{1+} and p_{+1} are free parameters and can be chosen to best fit the data set. In fact the best estimate is $\hat{p}_{1+} = 961/1841$ and $\hat{p}_{+1} = 1063/1841$, which leads to $1841\,\hat{p}_{1+}\hat{p}_{+1} = 554.9$ for the fitted value in this cell of the table.

Once the problem has been set in the well-known framework of parametric statistical inference, the procedures of maximum likelihood estimation and likelihood ratio tests are made available.

Extensions

The deep roots in probability and statistical theory ensure that the notions of graphical modelling easily generalize in two directions that enlarge the scope of applications: to variables that are continuous or mixed discrete and continuous, and to variables that embody response-explanatory structure. For continuous variables the natural measure of interaction is the correlation coefficient and the appropriate conditional measure is the partial correlation coefficient. The natural family of distributions is the multivariate normal distribution and the ensuing graphical models are called graphical Gaussian models. The family of mixed graphical models is based on an extension to the conditionally Gaussian distribution, which is rich enough to include linear and logistic regression as special cases.

A response explanatory structure is created by dividing the variables into two blocks: the response set $(R_1, R_2, \ldots, R_q)$ and the explanatory set $(E_1, E_2, \ldots, E_q)$. A combined model can be based on three types of tests:

(a) tests for the conditional independence of $E_i \perp\!\!\!\perp E_j \mid$ (rest of the Es) where the response variables are ignored
(b) tests for the conditional independence of $R_i \perp\!\!\!\perp R_j \mid$ (rest of the Rs and all the Es) where the explanatory variables are included
(c) tests for the conditional independence of $R_i \perp\!\!\!\perp E_j \mid$ (rest of the Rs and rest of the Es) where the explanatory variables are included.

To reflect the different types of independence statement, lines are used for intrablock edges (within the explanatory sets (a) and within the response set (b)) and arrows are used for interblock edges between the response and the explanatory variables (c). For example,

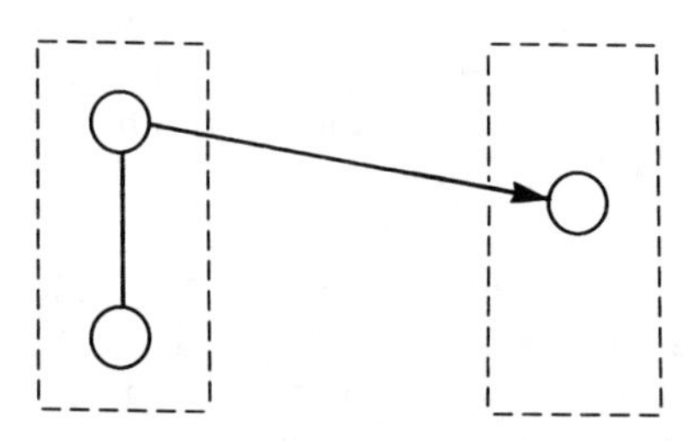

The technique can be generalized from two blocks to several blocks, giving rise to the chain graphs for more complicated patterns of dependence discussed by Wermuth in Chapter 9.

Practical Issues in Graphical Modelling

The notion of conditional independence and its associated independence graph makes rapid analysis of high-dimensional contingency tables possible. The directly computable array of edge exclusion deviances immediately characterizes the pattern of interaction between the variables that classify the table. The graph indicates any further possibility of reduction in dimension and focuses attention on highly interactive relationships. However, there are practical matters in the applications of these techniques to data analysis that have to be addressed: choice of variables, choice of response and explanatory variables, model selection, model fitting with sparse data, and diagnostic procedures.

There is no reason to suppose that conditioning on a particular set of variables is necessarily right. For example it could be that there is a subset of variables which are completely independent but are correlated with another variable; by conditioning on this variable as well, the independence in the subset is obscured. The following graph illustrates this, with the marginal distribution of (1, 2, 3) represented in the box:

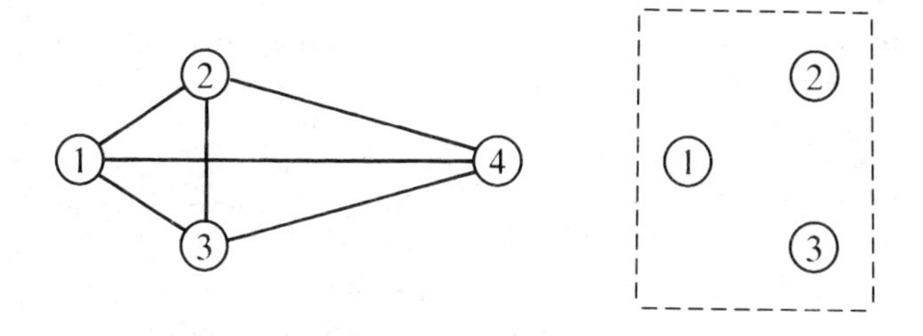

Or, to give an example in the opposite direction, there may be a superset of variables with a particularly simple independence graph, but, because no information is given on some variables, the graph of the observed variables is complicated. Here the unobserved superset is portrayed on the right:

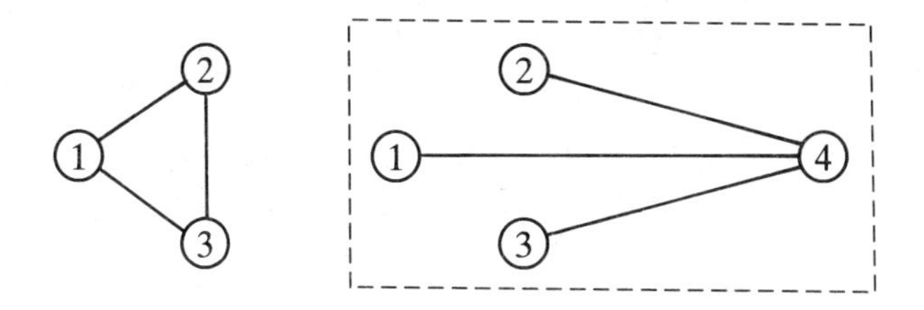

This is essentially a scientific issue, and it is up to the research investigator to isolate an interesting and a complete set of variables for study.

In a graph for k variables there are $\binom{k}{2}$ edges, and consequently $2^{\binom{k}{2}}$ different graphs to represent the data. Even for moderate k this is too large a figure to allow the examination of all possible models, but fortunately there are now fairly sophisticated model selection routines available similar to those for the related problem of variable selection in multiple regression analysis.

Sparse Tables

A statistical concern often arises because of the possible analysis of sparse tables. For example, consider the two-way Table 8.7. Because of the 0 entry in the total category for the $X = 2$ margin there is no information here to decide for or against the independence of X and Y. Even if the zeros are replaced by 1 and 2 say, giving a table based on six observations, the small number of observations makes the chi-squared distribution a very poor approximation to the distribution of the statistic when the null hypothesis is true. That is, the stated p-values may differ by several orders of magnitude from the true ones.

This situation is exacerbated when testing for conditional independence which, as noted above, examines independence in sets of two-way tables corresponding to slicing on the conditioning variables, and it is much more likely that there will be zeros or at least small values in these subtables. The price of examining multivariate interactions is the explosion of parameters that require estimating and in consequence the larger sample sizes needed to attain reasonable efficiencies. Further, the conditional independence tests are combined tests based on several degrees of freedom. Because of the unspecified nature of the departure from independence, it is likely that the power properties of the test are poor and that the procedure may not detect small but significant deviations from independence.

There are several remedies to these difficulties. Rather than depend on the large-sample approximation to the distribution of the test, it is possible to use an exact distribution which, though hard to tabulate, can be applied via simulation. This can result in dramatic

Table 8.7 *Another fictitious two-way table*

	$Y = 1$	$Y = 2$	Total
$X = 1$	1	2	3
$X = 2$	0	0	0
Total	1	2	3

improvements. The power may also be improved if the number of parameters can be reduced. For example, rather than test each slice against any departure from independence, test each against a common departure in each slice. Use of such techniques is discussed in Whittaker (1990: Chapter 8).

Finally, though there is no reason for the graph to be particularly simple, and in some applications with a moderate number of variables the missing edges appear to be haphazardly scattered over the graph (the spaghetti phenomenon), graphical modelling often does uncover simple patterns.

Latent Variable Diagrams and Conditional Independence Graphs

A latent variable is one that may not be observed directly and for which measurements can only be inferred from values of observed covariables. Measurement error models where all variables are subject to error and only approximate their true values provide one instance of latent variable modelling; factor analysis is another. In all they form an important subclass of statistical models, especially relevant in the health and social sciences. A good introduction is the book by Bartholomew (1987) (see also Arminger in Chapter 10 in this volume), and for a practical implementation see Jöreskog and Sörbom (1989). Parts of the literature stress the hidden variable aspect; others are more concerned with structural equations in latent variables, for example Bollen (1989).

It is often the case that the explication of a latent variable (LV) model is accompanied by a diagram which has very many similarities to the conditional independence (CI) graph; and the exact relationship between the graph and the diagram requires some puzzling out. Here we do so in the context of a specific combined regression-factor analysis model. The rules by which LV diagrams are constructed are not explicitly the same as those for CI graphs, so that *a priori* one might expect different pictures with different meanings. However, the relationship is sufficiently close to establish that, with some relatively minor modifications, certain LV diagrams can be interpreted as CI graphs and thereby enjoy the Markov properties of the CI graphs that make the latter so easily interpretable.

First, there are some distinctive features of LV diagrams to consider. Take for example the diagram of the combined regression-factor model, where three responses y_1, y_2 and y_3 are imagined to depend on explanatory variables x_1 and x_2 through the intervention of two latent variables or factors η_1 and η_2, as in the

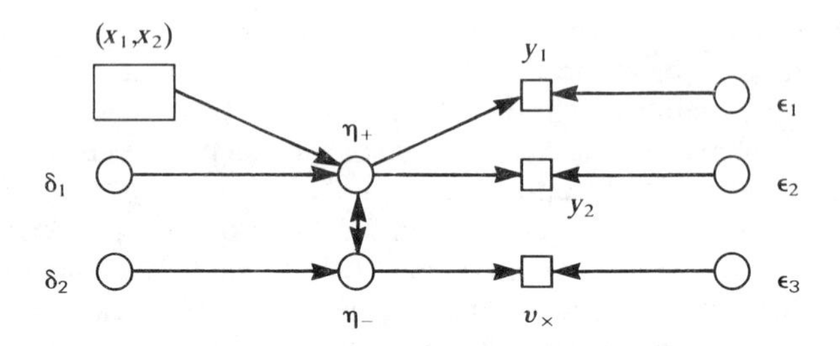

Figure 8.2 *An LV diagram for a combined regression-factor model*

LV diagram in Figure 8.2. To set a context: it might be that x_1 and x_2 measure smoking and alcohol intake, that y_1 and y_2 are independent measures of true blood pressure η_1, and that η_2 is a true lipid measure while y_3 is an indicator of that measure. Also suppose that the model is to be estimated from a survey of individuals. The ϵs and δs represent errors of measurement. The node is a box if the variable is observed and a circle if it is unobserved.

The LV diagram clarifies the structure of the model, but of course it is not a substitute for the detailed mathematical relations between the variables. Suppose the LV structure is such that the first factor η_1 depends on the exogenous regression variables x_1 and x_2 through the equation

$$\eta_1 = \beta_1 x_1 + \beta_2 x_2 + \gamma_2 \eta_2 + \delta_1$$

which incorporates a term in η_2 to model a correlation between the latent variables η_1 and η_2. The second variable η_2 does not depend on the explanatory variables directly, but is correlated with η_1; the equation is

$$\eta_2 = \gamma_1 \eta_1 + \delta_2$$

The observed variables depend on the latent variables through the observation equation

$$\begin{bmatrix} y_1 \\ y_2 \\ y_3 \end{bmatrix} = \begin{bmatrix} \lambda_1 & 0 \\ \lambda_2 & 0 \\ 0 & \lambda_3 \end{bmatrix} \begin{bmatrix} \eta_1 \\ \eta_2 \end{bmatrix} + \begin{bmatrix} \epsilon_1 \\ \epsilon_2 \\ \epsilon_3 \end{bmatrix}$$

The λs, the βs and the γs are fixed but unknown parameters, common to every subject in the survey, and need to be estimated. The errors δ and ϵ are assumed to be independent normally distributed random variables with variances σ_η^2 and σ_y^2, which, by the linearity of the equations in this example, imply that the observations have a multivariate normal distribution conditionally on the explanatory variables (though this is an unnecessarily restrictive assumption and can be generalized).

This joint distribution holds the independence structure of the full set of variables, and thereby of any marginal subset, and thus the information to determine the CI graph. How close is the LV diagram to the CI graph? First, there are some distinctive features of LV diagrams to consider. The distinction that observed variables have nodes marked as squares and unobserved variables have circles is not absolute, and from the point of view of probability each node has the same footing.

There is one problem with LV diagrams that relates to formations such as

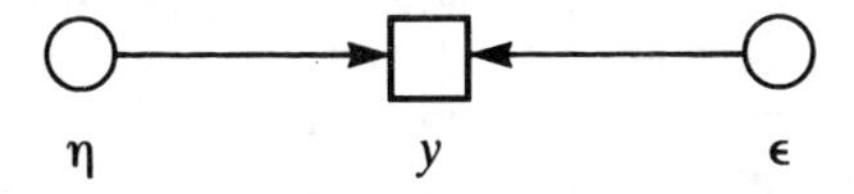

where $y = \eta + \epsilon$ and for which $\eta \perp\!\!\!\perp \epsilon$. Interpreted as a CI graph, this graph refers to the joint distribution of (y, η, ϵ) since these three vertices occur. But because of the linear relationship the joint distribution of these three variables is singular (degenerate). While this is not an insurmountable problem, some of the Markov properties fail to hold, in particular the pairwise Markov property. The easiest route is to redraw the diagram so as to exclude the error variables. Nothing is lost since these can all be computed from linear combinations of the observed and latent variables.

The diagram becomes Figure 8.3. This diagram is now an instance of the more general chain independence graph (which allows a mixture of directed and undirected edges). This is discussed by Wermuth in Chapter 9, and is closely related to a directed independence graph (influence diagram or conditional probability

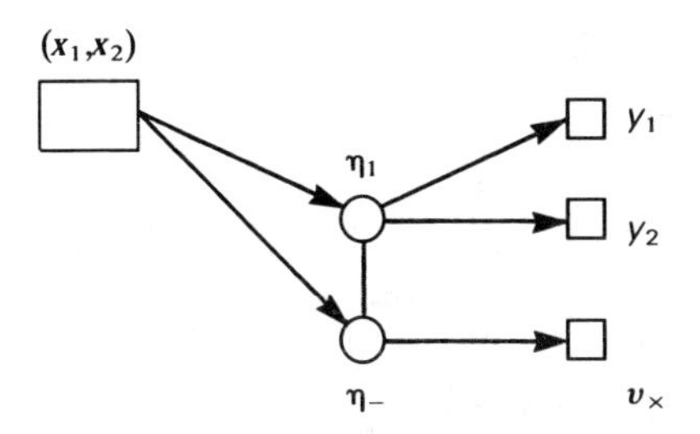

Figure 8.3 *The CI graph for the combined regression-factor model*

network). The nodes represent the variables or subsets of them, and the absence of edges expresses conditional independence relationships, where the directed edges indicate the conditioning set for the relationships. It can be directly verified from the joint distribution of the (y, η) given x that the following conditional independence statements are satisfied:

Structural independence $(y_1, y_2, y_3) \perp\!\!\!\perp (x_1, x_2) \mid (\eta_1, \eta_2)$ corresponding to the absence of directed edges from the x variables directly to the y variables.
Thurstone simple structure For each variable y_i there is an η_j such that $y_i \perp\!\!\!\perp \eta_{\text{rest}} \mid \eta_j$, so any y depends on one latent variable at most, as is easily evident from the diagram (or graph) where any response node has only one edge to the latent variables.
Local independence y_1, y_2, y_3 mutually $\perp\!\!\!\perp \mid (\eta_1, \eta_2)$ corresponding to the absence of any direct connection between the observed responses.

The chain graph has three blocks corresponding to the explanatory variables, the latent variables and the observed response variables. The analysis may equally well presume that the xs are fixed or random since the parameters of interest relate to the conditional distribution of (y, η) given x.

The acute reader will wonder at the induced edge between (x_1, x_2) and η_2. This occurs because the double-headed arrow in Figure 8.2 does not exactly translate to the undirected edge between η_1 and η_2 in Figure 8.3. A similar example, see Whittaker (1990: 302), would occur if the links between the latent variables and the explanatory variables are

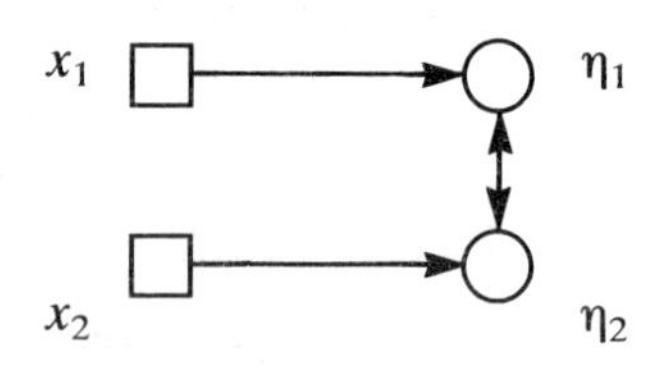

Then the fact that η_1 does not depend on x_2 and η_2 does not depend on x_1 in the LV diagram and model implies (using the corresponding structural equations) that

$$\eta_1 \perp\!\!\!\perp x_2 \mid x_1 \quad \text{and} \quad \eta_2 \perp\!\!\!\perp x_1 \mid x_2.$$

However, this neither implies nor is implied by

$$\eta_1 \perp\!\!\!\perp x_2 \mid (x_1, \eta_2) \quad \text{and} \quad \eta_2 \perp\!\!\!\perp x_1 \mid (x_2, \eta_1)$$

and it is these latter conditions that are needed for the CI graph.

From this description it can be seen that the latent variable diagram has a very intimate relationship with the associated directed CI graph, with the corollary that LV modelling is just a form of graphical modelling that incorporates latent variables.

Though there are differences in the exact independence specifications of the model, the great divide in practice is whether to utilize latent variables or not. The debate has been fairly well aired and tends to concentrate on the possibility or otherwise of making direct measurements on the variables of interest. If this is not possible then latent variable modelling is the only recourse. However, there is a price to pay in that LV diagrams are no longer necessarily verifiable against data, and the independence structure of the LV modeller is a product of assumption rather than of empirical observation.

Summary and Concluding Remarks

Conditional independence is a powerful though hitherto neglected concept of probability theory which only in recent years has achieved true recognition of its merits. In this chapter we have shown how the concept deals with certain complexities arising in the design and analysis of health studies.

Graphical model search simplifies the complexity of high-dimensional contingency tables and generates an appropriate graphical interaction model as a description of the data. The technique has been illustrated by a six-way ($k = 6$) contingency table compiled from a survey relating to possible prognostic factors for coronary heart disease in a study of car workers from Czechoslovakia. The distribution of the subjects in the cells of the table, that is the balance of the table, affects the inferential procedure in attribution of cause and effect. Detailed examination of imbalance, or equivalently the interaction pattern in the table, is effected by fitting a graphical model. By example it was argued that analysis in the two-way marginal tables is inadequate and even misleading because such analyses do not allow for the possibility that an observed pairwise interaction may be explained by the interaction with a third variable. However, tests for pairwise independence may be modified to allow for potential interaction with other variables, and the full set of $k(k - 1)/2$ adjusted tests may be combined into a single picture by means of a graph, the conditional independence graph.

The graph is defined by the fact that pairs of variables that are not directly connected are conditionally independent given the remaining variables. The graph has certain important properties: it is Markov in the sense that (1) any pair of non-adjacent variables is independent given only the values of those variables that separate the pair; and (2) there is no better predictor for one variable from the others than those that are nearest neighbours in the graph. Consequently the graph succinctly represents the pattern of multivariate associations and dependencies which, embodied within a framework of statistical distributions, define a graphical interaction model.

Extensions to continuous variables and to mixed discrete and continuous variables were briefly suggested, and also to response and explanatory variables which include the special case of linear and logistic regression, and extend to chain graphs for more complicated patterns of dependence. The close relationship to latent variable and factor analysis models was alluded to in the final section.

References

Bartholomew, D.J. (1987) *Latent Variable Models and Factor Analysis*. London: Griffin.

Bollen, K.A. (1989) *Structural Equations with Latent Variables*. New York: Wiley.

Darroch, J.N., Lauritzen, S.L. and Speed, T.P. (1980) 'Markov fields and log linear interaction models for contingency tables', *Annals of Statistics*, 8: 522–39.

Dawid, A.P. (1979) 'Conditional independence in statistical theory (with discussion)', *Journal of the Royal Statistical Society, Series B*, 41 (1): 1–31.

Jöreskog, K.G. and Sörbom, D. (1989) *LISREL 7: A Guide to the Program and Applications*, 2nd edn. Chicago: SPSS.

Whittaker, J. (1990) *Graphical Models in Applied Multivariate Statistics*. Chichester: Wiley.

Wright, S. (1921) 'Correlation and causation', *Journal of Agricultural Research*, 20: 557–85.

Wright, S. (1923) 'The theory of path coefficients: a reply to Niles' criticism', *Genetics*, 8: 239–55.

9

Association Structures with Few Variables: Characteristics and Examples

Nanny Wermuth

Introduction

The usefulness of any graphical representation depends on the ease with which its implications can be deduced and on whether it has an unambiguous interpretation or not.

Graphical chain representations were suggested (Lauritzen and Wermuth, 1989) to represent complex association structures among variables which may be qualitative or quantitative. The word 'association' is used broadly to include both symmetric associations for variables treated on an equal footing and directed relations concerned with the dependence of a response on explanatory variables, sometimes called influences. Symmetric associations occur not only when there are no response variables at all, but also when some variables are joint responses or joint influences, or when they are joint intermediate variables in the sense of being responses to one set of variables and influences on another.

Figure 9.1 shows as an example one possible graphical chain representation for six variables. Variable A is a direct response to variables B, X and C and an indirect response to D, Y; variables B and X are joint intermediate variables; and C, Y and D are regarded only as influences on X, B, as well as on A via X, B.

The purpose of this chapter is to illustrate some of the essential features of graphical chain representations, and to relate them to more traditional formulations of models as well as to familiar tasks in analysing data. To this end we define chain graphs and mention some related distributional assumptions. We discuss differences between using a chain graph to characterize a statistical model or a substantive research hypothesis. We present reasons for analysing the associations among influences in addition to the type of dependence of responses on the explanatory variables. We explain why interaction effects known from analyses of variance models or, more generally, for regression models are not reflected in graphical

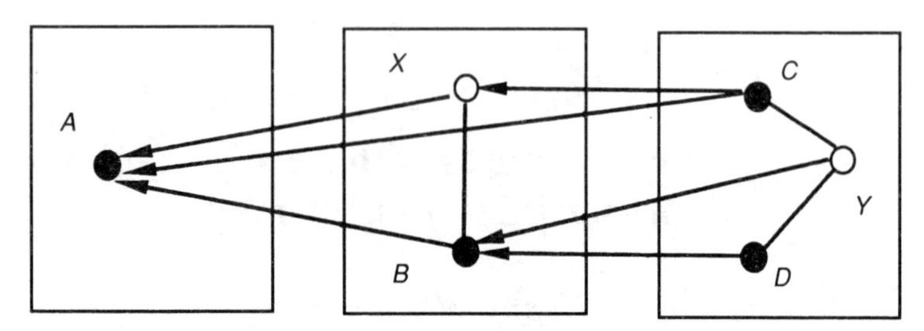

Figure 9.1 *Example of a graphical chain representation. A discrete variable* A *depends directly on the continuous variable* X *and on two discrete variables* B, C *and only indirectly on variables* Y *and* D. *The variables* X *and* B *are intermediate in the sense of being influences on variable* A *and joint responses to variables* C, D *and* Y, *while* C, D *and* Y *are regarded only as influences, that is explanatory variables*

chain representations. We illustrate the different types of analyses and chain graphs that can correspond to the familiar research question of whether a further explanatory variable will improve the prediction of a response. Finally, we discuss some relations of graphical chain models to linear structural relation models.

In this chapter the emphasis is on examples with few variables, but the theory has been developed for many variables. One of the main advantages of graphical chain representations is that problems with many variables which appear complex at first sight might be split up into a sequence of analyses, most of which involve far fewer variables.

Definition of Chain Graphs and Distributional Assumptions

The statistical models for the association structures that we consider consist of distributional assumptions and an independence structure, that is a set of independencies represented by a chain graph.

Chain Graphs

The chain graphs consist of points for variables, and of at most one line or one arrow as the connection of a variable pair, and can be arranged to form a chain of boxes. The chain structure has to be supplied from subject-matter knowledge about responses and potential influences. A chain graph drawn with boxes is viewed as a substantive research hypothesis (Wermuth and Lauritzen, 1990) about direct and indirect relations among variables and not only as a statistical model. In a graph of a statistical model, that is one drawn without boxes, a connected variable pair just means an unrestricted association, while in a graph of a substantive research hypothesis it stands for a non-vanishing association.

Points represent two types of property of observational units: variables with a nominal scale, called categorical or qualitative (drawn as dots); and variables for which numerical measurements are obtained, called quantitative (drawn as circles). There are two types of associations: the directed associations (drawn as arrows) for variable pairs, where one variable is regarded as a response and the other as an explanatory or influencing variable; and the symmetric associations (drawn as lines without arrowheads), where no direction of dependence has been specified.

If instead the graph just represents a statistical model, that is it is drawn without boxes, then such a model is defined for sets of discrete (dots) and continuous (circles) random variables in terms of specific distributional assumptions and a set of conditional independence restrictions. The graph depicts the independencies, since the set of missing direct connections for variable pairs corresponds to a specific conditional independence structure.

The convention adopted for the chain models of Lauritzen and Wermuth (1989) to ensure an unambiguous interpretation of each pairwise relation is that the conditioning variables of each pair are the remaining 'concurrent variables'. In graphs with dashed lines and arrows of multivariate regression chains (Wermuth and Cox, 1992a) – not discussed here – a different convention is used. The set of concurrent variables is obtained for a given pair (U, V) by ignoring all variables, to which *U and V* are potential influences, that is it is found by deleting from the picture all those boxes to which arrows from both U and V could point. In Figure 9.1, for example, the concurrent variables to (A, Y) are all six variables; to (X, Y) are all variables except A; and to (C, D) are C, D and Y.

Thus the missing link between C and D means conditional independence of C and D given Y $(C \perp D \mid Y)$; the missing arrow between B and C says that (B, C) is conditionally independent given X, D, Y $(B \perp C \mid (X, D, Y))$; the arrow from Y to B means a dependence of B on Y given X, C, D; the line between X and B represents a symmetric association between (X, B) given C, Y, D; and the single response A is conditionally independent of the indirect influences D, Y given the directly related explanatory variables B, X and C, that is $A \perp (D, Y) \mid (B, X, C)$.

This last independence statement is derived from the pairwise independencies and is one application of a result for general chain graphs by which one can read off the graph *all* implied independencies (Frydenberg, 1990). Though this result is most important for understanding and interpreting complex structures, it is less needed for the structures with few variables considered in this chapter.

Distributional Assumptions

The joint density fv in a graphical chain model can be expressed in terms of densities for the different sets of the concurrent variables, for instance for Figure 9.1 as

$$fv = f_{a|bc} f_{b|c} f_c \tag{9.1}$$

where $a=\{A\}$, $b=\{X,B\}$, $c=\{C,Y,D\}$ are called the elements of the dependence chain $\boldsymbol{C} = (a,b,c)$, and with three sets of concurrent variables $a \cup b \cup c$, $b \cup c$ and c. In principle a large number of different distributions corresponding to different special assumptions about the factors determining fv can belong to a chain graph; however, algorithms for estimating associations and for testing independencies are at present not available for many.

In the examples discussed here we assume conditional Gaussian (CG) distribution and regressions (Lauritzen and Wermuth, 1989). Special cases are as follows. For a single continuous response a CG regression can be a linear regression, an analysis of variance, or an analysis of covariance; for a single discrete response it is a linear or a quadratic logistic regression. A CG distribution takes the continuous variable to have a joint normal distribution conditional in each cell defined by the level combinations of the discrete variables; it leads to log-linear models if there are no continuous variables and to a joint normal distribution if there are no discrete variables.

Other distributional assumptions are possible. Some results of how such different assumptions will affect estimation and test results are available (Cox and Wermuth, 1992a).

Substantive Research Hypotheses versus Statistical Models

It can be helpful to distinguish between a statistical model represented by a chain graph drawn without boxes and a substantive research hypothesis represented by a chain graph drawn with boxes. A substantive research hypothesis depends strongly on subject-matter knowledge. Such knowledge typically involves not only indirect relations (modelled in connection with chain graphs via missing direct links which mean independencies) but also the relative strength and the type of associations among variables. In fact, the aim of much substantive research is to establish evidence for relations which are rather strong as compared to weak and

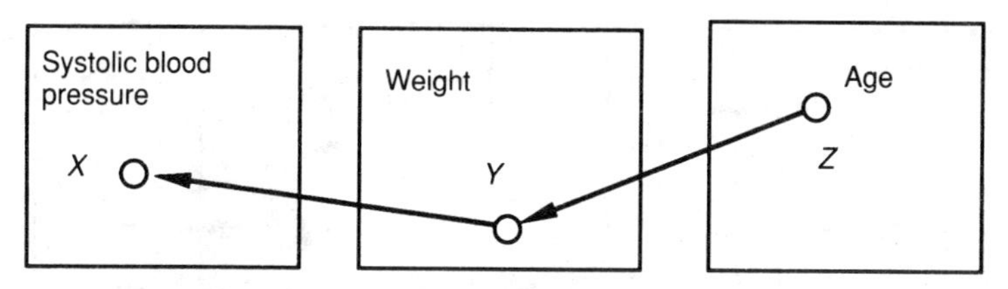

Figure 9.2 *Example for a simple substantive hypothesis: there is a non-vanishing dependence of systolic blood pressure* X *on weight* Y *and of weight* Y *on age* Z; X *is conditionally independent of* Z *given* Y (X ⊥ Z | Y), *that is systolic blood pressure* X *depends only indirectly on age* Z *since it is independent of age given information on weight* Y.

negligible ones. This is reflected in the graphical representation, that is connections in chain graphs drawn with boxes mean non-vanishing associations.

In contrast a statistical model for associations can be defined and studied without connection to any specific substantive issues. In it a relation between a variable pair is either restricted by an independence statement and gives a missing direct link in the chain graph, or regarded as unrestricted, that is permitted to vary freely within the limits specified by distributional assumptions.

For instance, for patients with hypertension, strong positive linear dependencies of systolic blood pressure X on both degree of overweight Y and age Z are expected, and a plausible hypothesis is that the dependence on age becomes rather unimportant given the information on degree of overweight. This substantive research hypothesis is expressed with the graph in Figure 9.2. It says that there is a non-negligible correlation between overweight and age (ρ_{yz}), and between systolic blood pressure and overweight (ρ_{xy}), but that knowing the age of a patient does not improve prediction of the degree of hypertension provided the information on degree of overweight is available ($\rho_{xz.y} = 0$). This research hypothesis implies in particular that the simple correlation ρ_{xz} of blood pressure and age is non-zero but is less strong than the smaller of ρ_{yz} and ρ_{xy}, since $\rho_{xz.y} = 0$ implies $\rho_{xz} = \rho_{yz}\rho_{xy}$ and correlations are smaller than one.

In contrast to the research hypothesis, the statistical model underlying Figure 9.2, which could have been specified as a trivariate normal distribution with $\rho_{xz.y} = 0$, does not imply a non-zero marginal association ρ_{xz}. In fact, it is consistent with either or both of ρ_{yz} and ρ_{xy} being zero, in which case ρ_{xz} would also be zero. All that can be derived from the statistical model is that $\rho_{xz} = 0$ is

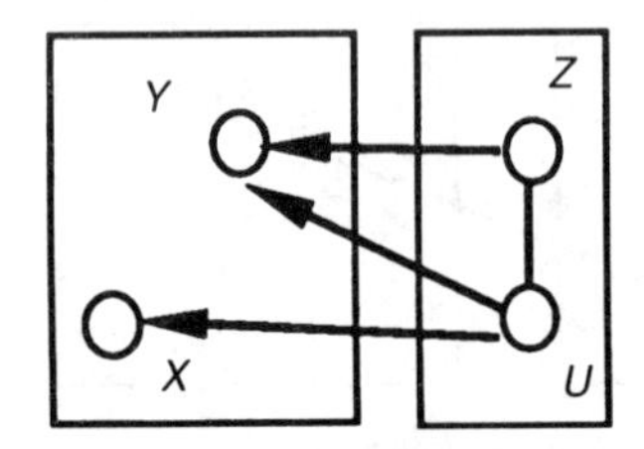

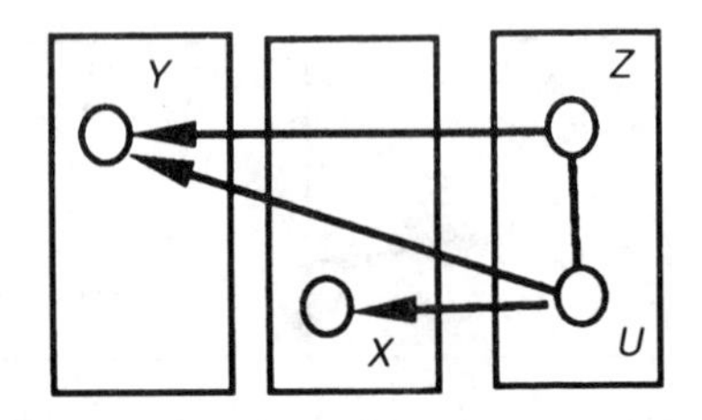

Figure 9.3 *Two distinct research hypotheses which correspond to the same statistical model; the missing edge* (X,Z) *means* $X \perp Z \mid (Y,U)$ *in the left graph and* $X \perp Z \mid U$ *in the right graph; the missing edge between* X *and* Y *means* $X \perp Y$ (Z,U), *in both graphs. A compact description of the set of independencies is* $X \perp (Y,Z) \mid U$ *in both graphs*

not implied, that is marginal independence of X and Z is not implied. This is a much weaker implication than the one derived from the research hypothesis.

It may also happen that several research hypotheses are compatible with the same statistical model. One example is given in Figure 9.3. In the left graph Z and U are potential joint influences on the joint responses X and Y, while in the right graph X is regarded as a potential influence on Y as well. Consequently, the meaning of pairwise relations can differ: for instance, the arrow from U to X is a dependence given Y and Z in the left graph, while it is a dependence given Z in the right graph.

To understand the meaning of a research hypothesis, it is crucial to know the dependence chain, since it assigns a specific meaning to each pairwise relation. This is not the case for the corresponding conditional independence structure since it depends only on the underlying chain graph (Frydenberg, 1990). A chain graph used to characterize a statistical model can be obtained from a graph characterizing a research hypothesis by deleting the boxes, that is by ignoring the specific ordering of the variables given in terms of a dependence chain.

The data in Table 9.1 for 98 healthy male adults (Hodapp et al., 1988) show that the research hypothesis of Figure 9.2 is also compatible with observations for persons not suffering from hypertension. The observed partial correlation $r_{xz.y}$ is almost zero and the marginal correlations are all positive, though the strength of the correlations for this collective of healthy persons is smaller than expected for a collective of hypertensive patients.

No statistical test could have rejected the hypothesis $\rho_{xz} = 0$, since the observed correlation is rather small ($r_{xz} = 0.139$). How-

Table 9.1 *Risk factors for cardiovascular diseases: observed marginal correlations (lower half), observed partial correlations (upper half) and further data summaries, n=98*

Variable	*X* Systolic blood pressure	*Y* Weight	*Z* Age
X Systolic blood pressure	1	0.348	−0.007
Y Weight relative to height	0.371	1	0.369
Z Age	0.139	0.390	1
Mean	128.31	0.42	32.74
Standard deviation	13.47	0.04	11.67

ever, it would be unwise to use such a test and its result in the present context: it would mean to ignore the available subject-matter knowledge, in particular the implication of the research hypothesis in Figure 9.2.

Reasons for Analysing Relations among Explanatory Variables

If observations become available from a particular study, there will be expectations on the part of the investigator regarding strength, direction or lack of associations not only for the response variables but also for the potential explanatory variables. This alone is an important reason to investigate relations among explanatory variables.

If unexpected findings are encountered there may be systematic errors in the data or there may be selection effects. For instance, in a study of effects of different pre-operative sedative treatments an unexpected strong association between vigilance, a strategy to cope with anxiety and stress, and gender of patients was observed. The reason for this turned out to be a selection strategy: the anaesthetist had allocated to the control group, that is to no pre-operative treatment at all, only those patients who appeared to be least excited. As a consequence, patients in the control group had characteristics quite distinct from patients in treated groups.

Another important reason for analysing relations among explanatory variables is to investigate whether moderation in the confounding sense (Breslow and Day, 1980; Wermuth, 1992a) can be a feature of the investigated relations. This means that an association which coincides in several subgroups is qualitatively different overall, that is without a split into subgroups. In the literature on

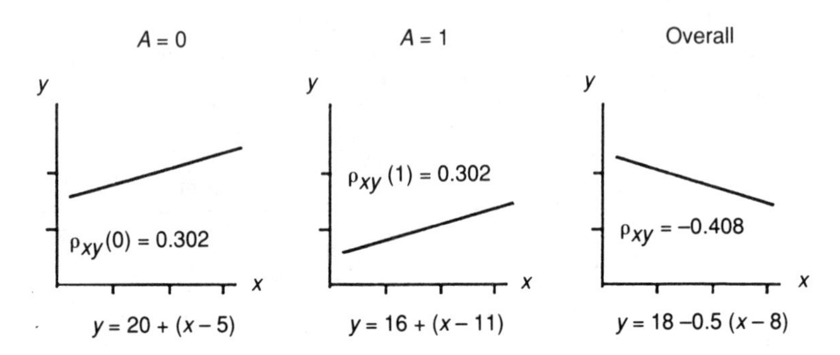

Figure 9.4 *Example for moderation in the confounding sense with:* $\mu_y(0) = 20$, $\mu_x(0) = 5$, $\sigma_{yy}(0) = 11$, $\sigma_{xx}(0) = 1$, $\sigma_{xy}(0) = 1$; $\mu_y(1) = 16$, $\mu_x(1) = 11$, $\sigma_{yy}(1) = 11$, $\sigma_{xx}(1) = 1$, $\sigma_{xy}(1) = 1$; *and* $Pr(A = 0) = Pr(A = 1) = 0.5$

contingency tables, such situations have been called the Yule-Simpson paradox (Simpson, 1951; Wermuth, 1989). A particularly striking version of it is shown for parallel linear regressions in Figure 9.4.

Moderation in the confounding sense is further illustrated with fictitious data for a contingency table in Table 9.2. A reversal in the direction of dependence after marginalizing over one of the explanatory variables cannot occur with independent explanatory variables; it is more likely the stronger the explanatory variables are associated. It is most important to be aware of moderation in the confounding sense if results from two studies are to be compared; confounding can be the explanation for results which appear contradictory at first sight.

Chain Graphs and Interactions

A missing link in a chain graph means a conditional independence, and a direct connection between a variable pair means a particular – not further specified – conditional association. For purposes of interpretation it is important to understand how these concepts relate to more traditional definitions of interactions.

Fisher (for example, 1956: Chapter 42) had introduced interaction in a two-way analysis of variance context to mean a different dependence of the response on one explanatory variable for different levels of the second variable, that is as a two-factor interaction in a model for dependence of a quantitative response X on two qualitative explanatory variables A and B. X had a normal distribution given A and B, possibly differing in means but not in

Table 9.2 *Examples with strongly consistent results within sites in terms of relative risks, which have value 1.5 at each site, and appear reversed overall in case (a) but are replicated in case (b)*

(a) Yule-Simpson paradox (moderation in the confounding sense)

Outcome	Clinic X: treatment A	Clinic X: treatment B	Clinic O: treatment A	Clinic O: treatment B	Overall: treatment A	Overall: treatment B
1	600 (30%)	40 (20%)	300 (75%)	2000 (50%)	900 (38%)	2040 (49%)
2	1400	160	100	2000	1500	2160
Sum	2000	200	400	4000	2400	4200
	$\frac{\pi_{1\mid AX}}{\pi_{1\mid BX}} = 1.5$		$\frac{\pi_{1\mid AO}}{\pi_{1\mid BO}} = 1.5$		$\frac{\pi_{1\mid A}}{\pi_{1\mid B}} = 0.78$	

(b) Relative risk is collapsible since explanatory variables are independent

Outcome	Clinic X: treatment A	Clinic X: treatment B	Clinic O: treatment A	Clinic O: treatment B	Overall: treatment A	Overall: treatment B
1	60 (30%)	400 (20%)	300 (75%)	2000 (50%)	360 (60%)	2400 (40%)
2	140	1600	100	2000	240	3600
Sum	200	2000	400	4000	600	6000
	$\frac{\pi_{1\mid AX}}{\pi_{1\mid BX}} = 1.5$		$\frac{\pi_{1\mid AO}}{\pi_{1\mid BO}} = 1.5$		$\frac{\pi_{1\mid A}}{\pi_{1\mid B}} = 1.5$	

variance. Conditional independence of X of A given B can in this model be expressed as $g_{x|ij}^{X|AB} = g_{x|j}^{X|B}$, and implies that there is no main effect of A and no two-factor interaction of A, B on X.

These notions have been extended to other dependence models. For instance, for a linear regression of X on a quantitative influence Y and a qualitative influence A, a two-factor interaction of A, Y on X means changing slopes of the linear regressions of X on Y at the different levels of A; that is, the lack of a two-factor interaction implies parallel regressions. Conditional independence of the response X of A requires in addition that the main effect is missing. More precisely, $X \perp A \mid Y$ implies that the parallel regression lines coincide, that is have equal intercepts of all levels of A.

The same interpretation applies to other CG regressions, that is logistic regressions with qualitative explanatory variables $g_{i|jk}^{A|BC}$ or with mixed explanatory variables $g_{i|jx}^{A|BX}$, and also to corresponding probit regressions.

Bartlett (1935) had given a definition of a three-factor interaction in a three-dimensional contingency table: changing odds ratios of two variables for different levels of the third variable. Though this definition for log-linear models appears to be quite similar to Fisher's definition, there is the important distinction in that it concerns interaction in a joint distribution, that is in a model for symmetric associations, and not the more commonly considered interaction in models for dependencies (Cox, 1984).

Conditional independence of A of B given C in a long-linear model can be expressed as $g_{ijk}^{ABC} = g_{ik}^{AC} g_{jk}^{BC} / g_k^C$ and it implies in particular that there is no log-linear two-factor interaction of A, B and no three-factor interaction. Since $g_{i|jk}^{A|BC} = g_{ijk}^{ABC} / g_{jk}^{BC} = g_{i|k}^{A|C}$ there is a correspondence between missing one- and two-factor interactions (B, BC) in a regression of A on B, C and missing two- and three-factor interactions (AB, ABC) in a joint distribution: they are equivalent formulations for conditional independence of (A,B) given C.

Bartlett's notion of interaction in a joint distribution and its relation to interactions in corresponding regression models has been extended to other than log-linear models with CG distributions and corresponding CG regressions. In any CG distribution a variable pair is conditionally independent given all of the remaining variables if and only if the two-factor interaction and all higher-order interactions of this pair vanish. Furthermore, vanishing of two- and higher-order interactions in the joint distribution implies the vanishing of a main effect and higher-order interactions in a corresponding CG regression which has one variable of the pair as a univariate response. This gives the precise meaning of a missing line and of a missing arrow in a chain graph in terms of interactions.

Similarly, an arrow in a chain graph means the presence of a main effect *or* of a two-factor *or* of a higher-order interaction in a regression, and a line means the presence of a two-factor *or* of a higher-order interaction in a joint distribution. This explains why a graphical chain representation completely describes independencies but only incompletely specifies the type of associations which are present. To give an example we take the symmetric association structure for three symptoms of EPH gestosis (Wermuth and Koller, 1976), an illness occurring during pregnancy, and symptoms after LSD intake (Lienert, 1970). The symptoms for the gestosis data are A yedema, B proteinuria and C hypertension, and for the LSD data they are distortions in: A thinking, B consciousness and C affective behaviour (Table 9.3).

In both cases the graphical chain representation is a complete graph with lines connecting all three symptom pairs. However, the

Table 9.3 *Counts for combinations of three symptoms of EPH gestosis and after LSD intake*

Data set	Symptom	Levels and counts							
	A	1	0	1	0	1	0	1	0
	B	1	1	0	0	1	1	0	0
	C	1	1	1	1	0	0	0	0
LSD intake[1]		21	4	2	11	5	16	13	1
EPH gestosis		14	9	36	45	26	44	609	2342

[1] One observation has been added to each cell.

association structures are quite different in the two situations. There is no log-linear three-factor interaction for the gestosis data but a strong log-linear three-factor interaction for the LSD data. All two-way margins show strong associations for the EPH data, but rather weak associations for the LSD data. These differences are not captured in the graph. The graphs just reflect the conditioning sets for each substantial dependence or association and the conditional independencies if there are any. Thus they show, for large sets of variables, to which sequences of smaller problems the analysis may be simplified.

Prediction of a Response: Is It Improved by an Additional Explanatory Variable?

In many research situations in which past research has established the dependence of a response variable X on a single explanatory variable Y $(h_{x|y}^{X|Y} \neq h_x^X)$, a natural next question is whether prediction of the response might be further improved by another variable Z. If this is not the case we have $X \perp Z \mid Y$ or $h_{x|yz}^{X|YZ} = h_{x|y}^{X|Y}$, and hence, the type of dependence of X on Y is not moderated at all by Z. If, however, the response is dependent on the additional explanatory variables, it becomes necessary to describe the type of dependence; in particular, it can be an issue whether there is moderation in the interactional or in the confounding sense (Wermuth, 1992a). In the case of moderation in the confounding sense the direction of a dependence can appear reversed after a second variable is included in the regression. In the case of moderation in the interactional sense the dependence of the response on an explanatory variable differs with different levels of the other explanatory variable.

Quite different types of analyses are needed in such situations depending on whether the involved variables are qualitative or quantitative. We give three examples in Figure 9.5. In the first

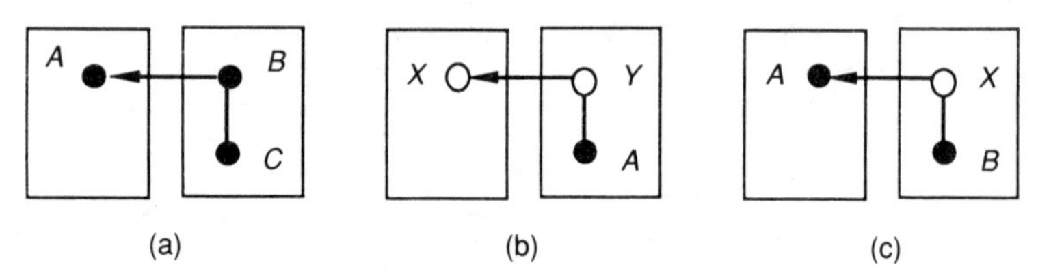

Figure 9.5 *Three regression chain graphs corresponding to the same type of research hypothesis: of two associated explanatory variables, only one is needed to predict the response.*
(a) Logistic regression chain with two qualitative explanatory variables; (b) linear regression chain with mixed explanatory variables; (c) logistic regression chain with mixed explanatory variables

example (Figure 9.5a) observations on n = 25,777 women (National Institutes of Health, 1972) are available for three qualitative variables A, B, C defined as follows:

A perinatal death (i = 1 yes; i = 2 no)
B survival state of last prior child (j = 1 living; j = 2 child death; j = 3 foetal death; j = 4 neonatal death; j = 5 unknown)
C skin colour of woman (k = 1 light; k = 2 dark).

The counts and the observed risks (in percentage rates) for perinatal mortality A at each of the level combinations of the potential influences B, C are given in Table 9.4. The research hypothesis is that prediction of the risk of perinatal mortality is not improved by the information on the skin colour of the mother provided a good indicator for the medical and socioeconomic situation of the mother is available. The test results in Table 9.5 and the mortality rates estimated under this hypothesis (Table 9.4) show how well the hypothesis is compatible with the observations. As a final summary the estimated relative risks for perinatal mortality are displayed in Table 9.4. The increase in risk for perinatal mortality as compared with the best condition (the last child prior to the present is alive) is substantial. The relative risk of 4.2, for instance, says that the risk for perinatal mortality is four times higher under the worst condition (survival status of last child unknown) as compared with the best condition. This risk increase due to poor socioeconomic conditions of the mother is higher than most risk increases owing to medical factors reported in National Institutes of Health (1972).

In the second example (Figure 9.5b) there are observations for n=40 patients prior to an operation on the jaw (Krohne et al., 1989). None of the patients have been treated with sedative drugs,

Table 9.4 *Counts and other data summaries for perinatal deaths (A), survival status of last prior child (B), and skin colour of woman (C)*

Levels			Observed	Observed	Estimates under $\pi_{i\|jk} = \pi_{i\|j}$		
A	*B*	*C*	count	% rate	Count	% rate	Relative risk
1	1	1	270	0.28	297.5	0.32	
2	1	1	9,148		9,120.5		
1	2	1	3	0.27	3.4	0.31	1
2	2	1	108		107.6		
1	3	1	134	0.74	132.8	0.73	2.3
2	3	1	1,678		1,679.2		
1	4	1	17	0.90	19.3	1.02	3.2
2	4	1	173		170.7		
1	5	1	56	1.26	59.3	1.33	4.2
2	5	1	389		385.7		
1	1	2	371	0.34	343.5	0.32	
2	1	2	10,502		10,529.5		
1	2	2	5	0.34	4.6	0.31	1
2	2	2	144		144.4		
1	3	2	154	0.72	155.2	0.73	2.3
2	3	2	1,963		1,961.8		
1	4	2	37	1.08	34.7	1.02	3.2
2	4	2	305		307.3		
1	5	2	46	1.44	42.7	1.33	4.2
2	5	2	274		277.3		

Source: National Institutes of Health, 1972: 187

Table 9.5 *Tests for conditional independencies, Table 9.4 data*

Pair	Concurrent variables	Values of chi-square statistic	Degrees of freedom	Corresponding fractile or *p*-value
(A,B)	*ABC*	279.12	8	<0.001
(A,C)	*ABC*	6.03	5	0.302
(B,C)	*BC*	68.81	4	<0.001

and – owing to a selection strategy of the anaesthetist – all have in common that they are non-vigilant, that is they do not use vigilant behaviour as a strategy in copying with stress. The variables are as follows:

X level of free fatty acids measured in the blood just before the operation

Table 9.6 *Effects of pre-operative anxiety Y on free fatty acids X*

	Overall		A=1		A=2	
	X	Y	X	Y	X	Y
Mean	390.8	41.7	434.8	44.0	346.7	39.5
Standard deviation	156.6	11.2	165.9	12.3	136.8	9.8
Correlation	0.38		0.54		0.06	
Number of patients	40		20		20	

Y level of anxiety measured with a state anxiety questionnaire on the morning of the day of the operation

A coping strategy 'cognitive avoidance' (1 = not employed; 2 = employed; categories were obtained by median dichotomizing the corresponding questionnaire scores U).

The research hypotheses are that either the coping strategy does not modify the dependence of free fatty acids on anxiety (as displayed in Figure 9.5b) or, if it does, a stronger dependence of physiological reaction on anxiety is expected if the patients do not use a strategy to cope with anxiety than if they do. When such a change in association is expected, any analysis based only on simple and partial correlations of the variables X, Y and U would not be suitable.

Table 9.6 gives the basic data summaries and Figure 9.6 shows the scatter plots between X and Y for A=1 and A=2, to ascertain that the observed changes in association between X and Y are not due to outliers or other irregularities of the data. Thus the data lead to a rejection of the hypothesis that information on the coping strategy is not needed to predict the level of free fatty acids from the level of anxiety. Instead the data support the described expectations regarding changes in associations, that is there is the expected interaction effect of Y and A on X.

In the third example (Figure 9.5c) the response variable is again qualitative, it is known to depend on a quantitative explanatory variable, and a potential qualitative moderator variable is considered. The observed variables for n=149 patients (Schmitt, 1990) are as follows:

A success of treatment (0 = no; 1 = yes) obtained from dichotomizing a more detailed score

X stage of chronic pain, a constructed indicator with possible values from 4 to 12

B gender.

In this context the hypothesis in Figure 9.5c says that the depen-

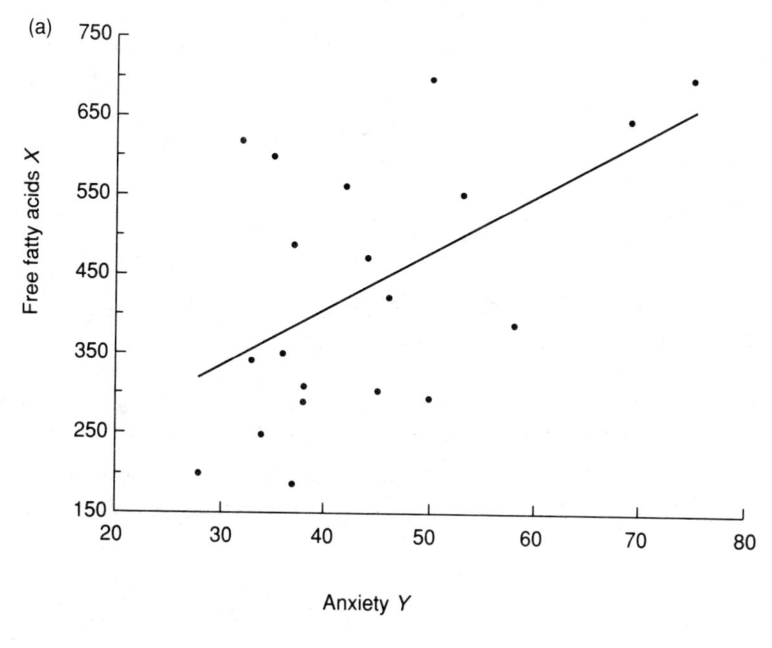

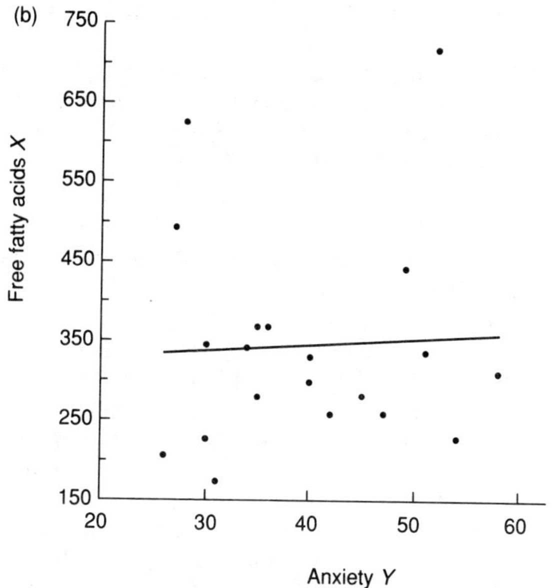

Figure 9.6 *Dependence of free fatty acids* X *on anxiety* Y *if the coping strategy of cognitive avoidance is (a) not employed (*A=*1) and (b) employed (*A = *2)*

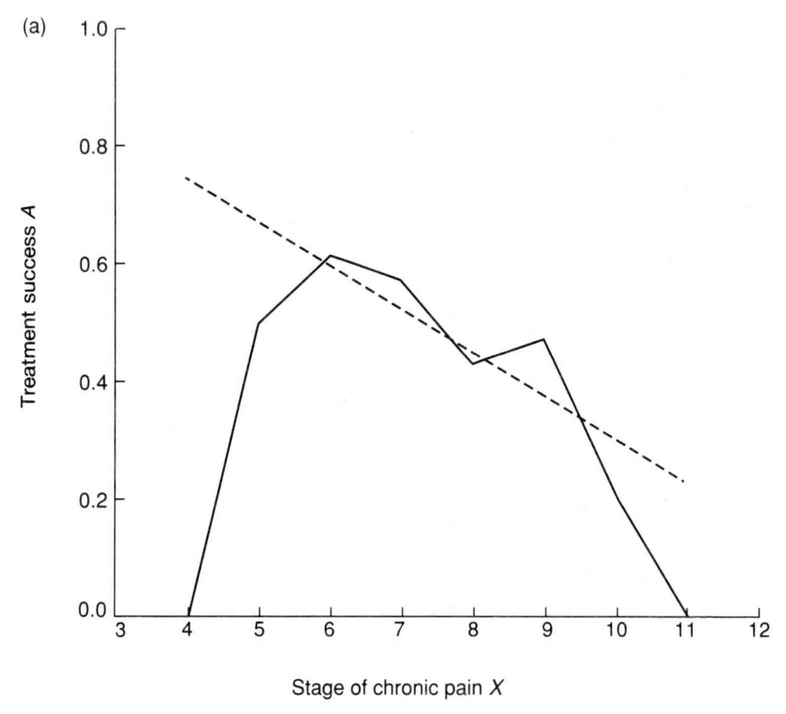

Figure 9.7 *Observed frequencies for success of treatment* A *as it depends on stage of chronic pain* X *and probabilities estimated by (a) linear logistic regression and (b) quadratic logistic regression. Solid line is smoothed observed values, broken lines are predictions*

dence of success of treatment on the stage of chronic pain is the same for males and females.

These data for a logistic regression provide one of the many examples in which an automatic search procedure leads to misleading results because the distributional assumptions in the research procedure amount to an overspecification; that is, if in this case the stepwise logistic regression of BMDP is used, which is a model search based only on global test statistics in linear logistic regression. More precisely, if one starts by assuming a linear logistic regression for X on Y it appears as if gender has no moderating effect on the dependence of success of treatment on stage of chronic pain. The computed goodness-of-fit statistics do not point to a bad fit of the models. This poor fit is, however, easily discovered from plotting fitted against observed probabilities of success as shown in Figure 9.7a.

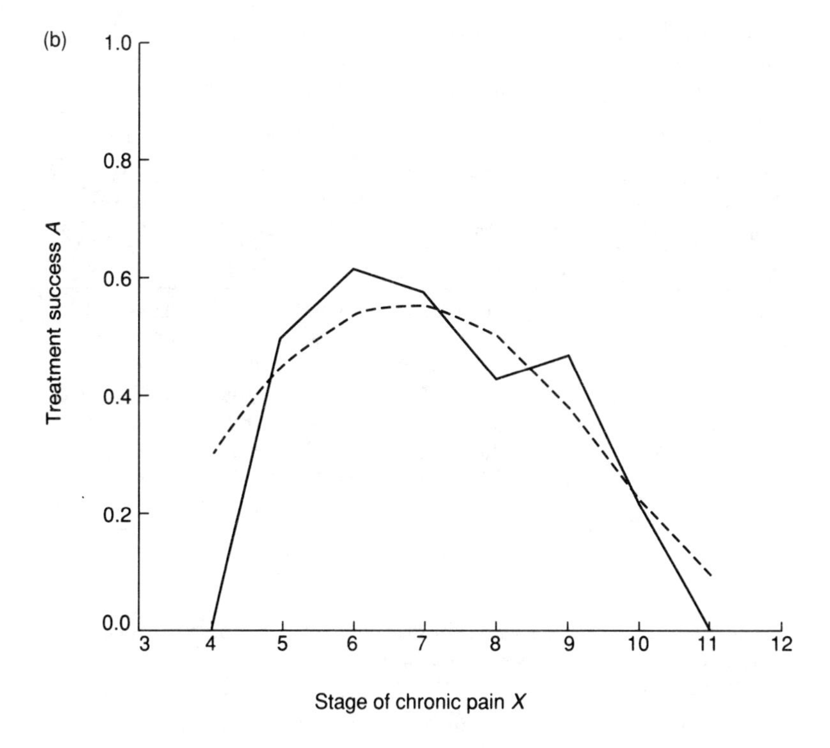

Figure 9.7 *continued*

If instead of assuming linear logistic regression we permit a quadratic dependence, that is we use the assumption of a non-homogeneous CG regression chain, then not only do we obtain a good fit overall as shown in Figure 9.7b, but gender emerges as an important moderator in the interactional sense. Observed and estimated success rates are displayed in Table 9.7 and in Figure 9.8. In this case the estimation results point to an unexpected interaction effect. It turns out that the patients with low success rates of treatment in spite of low scores for the stage of chronic pain are female headache patients. Further observations will be needed to judge the relevance of the result.

Relations to Other Models

Linear regressions and probit regressions are also assumptions used for models of linear structural relations (Jöreskog, 1977; Muthén, 1984). However, graphical representations of the latter cannot in

Table 9.7 *Scores for stage of chronic pain (X), counts, and estimated probabilities of success of treatment when leaving the clinic (A) for n = 149 patients given gender (B) and stage (X)*

					Probabilities estimated by:			
Stage of chronic pain	Total count		Number of successes		observed relative frequencies		quadratic logistic regression	
	Females	Males	Females	Males	Females	Males	Females	Males
x	$n_{.1x}$	$n_{.2x}$	n_{11x}	n_{12x}	$n_{1\mid 1x}$	$n_{1\mid 2x}$		
4	1	–	0	–	0.00	–	0.06	–
5	2	–	1	–	0.50	–	0.21	–
6	5	8	1	7	0.20	0.88	0.39	0.80
7	12	9	7	5	0.58	0.56	0.50	0.63
8	36	15	16	6	0.44	0.40	0.50	0.47
9	20	14	10	6	0.50	0.43	0.39	0.34
10	14	10	2	3	0.14	0.30	0.20	0.27
11	1	2	0	0	0.00	0.00	0.06	0.24

general be interpreted as chain graphs. One exception is when they correspond to systems of univariate recursive equations (see Wold, 1954; Wermuth and Lauritzen, 1983). Such graphs have been called univariate recursive (Wermuth and Lauritzen, 1990) or directed acyclic graphs (Pearl, 1988). Another exception is if they correspond to a multivariate regression or to a block-regression model (Wermuth, 1992b).

Models defined for univariate recursive systems within either framework, that is as a structural relation model or as a CG regression chain model, can be identical, similar or rather different. They are identical if all responses are continuous variables. They are rather similar if they only differ in probit versus logistic regression, since linear logistic regressions are virtually indistinguishable from linear probit regressions (Cox, 1966; Cox and Snell, 1989). They differ substantially if a quadratic logistic regression appears in the CG regression chain model but only a linear probit regression in the corresponding structural relation model.

There exist conditional independence structures which can be tested directly within the framework of graphical chain models but not within the framework of linear structural relations, and vice versa. A simple example of the former is displayed in Figure 9.9 and Table 9.8. An example for the latter is $X \perp U \mid Z$ *and* $Y \perp Z \mid U$, which can be interpreted as a hypothesis in a multivariate regression of X and Y on U and Z (see Cox and Wermuth, 1993).

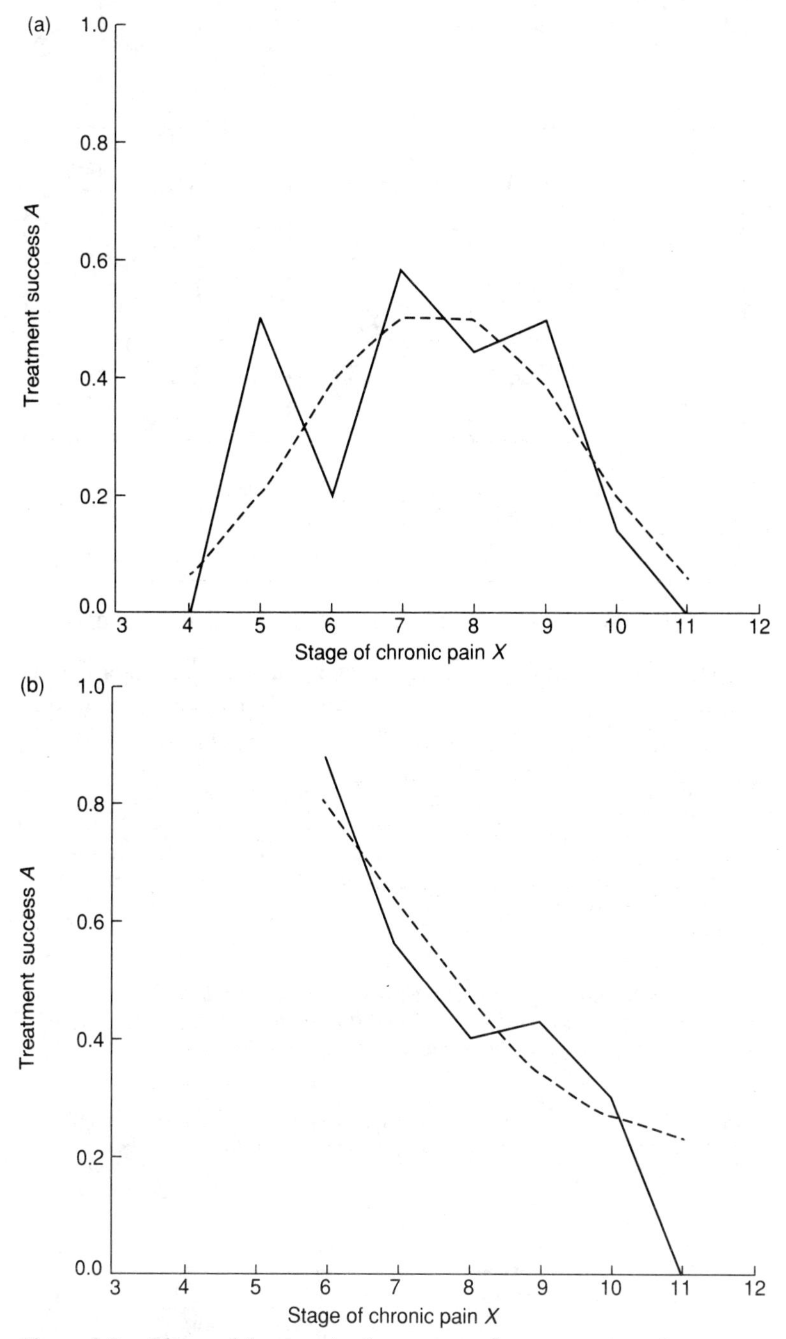

Figure 9.8 *Observed frequencies for success of treatment* A *and probabilities estimated by quadratic logistic regression given stage of chronic pain* X *and gender* B *for (a) females and (b) males. Solid line is smoothed observed values, broken lines are predictions*

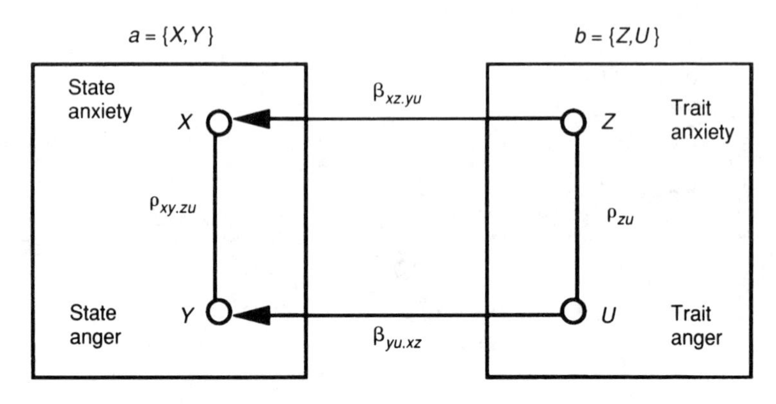

Figure 9.9 *A chain graph with a nondecomposable hypothesis:* X ⊥ U | (Y,Z) *and* Y ⊥ Z | (X,U)

The main disadvantages of linear structural equation models are:

1 The interpretation of each model, that is the meaning of parameters and of missing direct connections, has to be derived from scratch in most situations, since no general results are available to deduce them.
2 The meaning of equation parameters in linear structural relations is not tied to the notion of independence. It may, in particular, occur that by imposing one more zero restriction in a model, one suddenly has a situation in which some parameters are unidentifiable.

Table 9.8 *Observed marginal correlations (lower half) and observed partial correlations given all remaining variables (upper half), and further data summaries, n=684*

Variable	*X* State anxiety	*Y* State anger	*Z* Trait anxiety	*U* Trait anger
X State anxiety	1	0.45	0.47	– 0.04
Y State anger	0.61	1	0.03	0.32
Z Trait anxiety	0.62	0.47	1	0.32
U Trait anger	0.39	0.50	0.49	1
Mean	18.87	15.23	21.20	23.42
Standard deviation	6.10	6.70	5.68	6.57

Source: C.D. Spielberger, personal communication of data on anger, anxiety (1983).

3 A discrete variable enters as a response variable only by assuming an underlying normal variate which has been partitioned to give the categorized variable. This excludes nominal scaled variables and models for symmetric associations with three-factor interactions, that is explanations for data like those reported by Lienert (Table 9.3).

These disadvantages are not shared by graphical chain models. Their main disadvantages are of a different kind:

1 No programmed algorithms are widely available yet which permit the computation of estimates for each model in this class; such a development is likely to build on work by Frydenberg and Edwards (1989), Cox and Wermuth (1990; 1991) and Jensen et al. (1991).
2 The statistical theory for models with latent variables which is needed in many applications is not yet well developed.
3 More examples of good analyses with many variables would be helpful.

Though a considerable amount of new work on different special aspects of models for multivariate dependencies and associations has been published, for instance Cox and Wermuth (1992a; 1992b; 1992c; 1993) and Wermuth and Cox (1992a; 1992b; 1992c) much more needs to be done.

References

Bartlett, M.S. (1935) 'Contingency table interactions', *Supplement, Journal of the Royal Statistical Society*, 2: 248–52.

Breslow, N. and Day, N. (1980) *The Analysis of Case-Control Studies: Statistical Analysis in Cancer Research*. Lyon: International Agency for Research on Cancer.

Cox, D.R. (1966) 'Some procedures connected with the logistic qualitative response curve', in F.N. David (ed.), *Research Papers in Statistics: Essays in Honour of J. Neyman's 70th Birthday*. London: Wiley. pp. 55–71.

Cox, D.R. (1984) 'Interaction', *International Statistical Review*, 52: 1–31.

Cox, D.R. and Snell, E.J. (1989) *Analysis of Binary Data*, 2nd edn. London: Chapman and Hall.

Cox, D.R. and Wermuth, N. (1990) 'An approximation to maximum-likelihood estimates in reduced models', *Biometrika*, 77: 747–61.

Cox, D.R. and Wermuth, N. (1991) 'A simple approximation for bivariate and trivariate normal integrals', *International Statistical Review*, 59: 263–9.

Cox, D.R. and Wermuth, N. (1992a) 'Response models for mixed binary and quantitative variables', *Biometrika*, 79: 441–61.

Cox, D.R. and Wermuth, N. (1992b) 'On the calculation of derived variables in the analysis of multivariate responses', *Journal of Multivariate Analysis*, 42: 162–70.

Cox, D.R. and Wermuth, N. (1992c), 'A comment on the coefficient of determination for binary responses', *American Statistician*, 46: 1–4.

Cox, D.R. and Wermuth, N. (1993) 'Linear dependencies represented by chain-graphs.' To appear with discussion in *Statistical Science*.

Fisher, R.A. (1956) *Statistische Methoden für die Wissenschaft*, 12th edn. Edinburgh: Oliver and Boyd.

Frydenberg, M. (1990) 'The chain graph Markov property', *Scandinavian Journal of Statistics*, 17: 333–54.

Frydenberg, M. and Edwards, D. (1989) 'A modified iterative proportional scaling algorithm for estimation in regular exponential families', *Computational Statistics and Data Analysis*, 8: 143–53.

Hodapp, V., Neuser, K.W. and Weyer, G. (1988) 'Job stress, emotion, and work environment: toward a causal model', *Personality and Individual Differences*, 9: 851–9.

Jensen, S.T., Johansen, S. and Lauritzen, S.L. (1991) 'Globally convergent algorithms for maximizing a likelihood function', *Biometrika*, 78: 867–78.

Jöreskog, K.G. (1977) 'Structural equation models in the social sciences: specification, estimation and testing', in P.R. Krishnaiah (ed.), *Applications of Statistics*. Amsterdam: North-Holland. pp. 267–87.

Krohne, H.W., Kleemann, P.P., Hardt, J. and Theisen, A. (1989) 'Beziehungen zwischen Bewältigungsstrategien und präoperativen Streßreaktionen', *Zeitschrift für Klinische Psychologie*, 18: 350–64.

Lauritzen, S.L. and Wermuth, N. (1989) 'Graphical models for associations between variables, some of which are qualitative and some quantitative', *Annals of Statistics*, 17: 31–57.

Lienert, G.A. (1970) 'Konfigurationsfrequenzanalyse einiger Lysergsäure-diäthylamid-Wirkungen', *Arzneimittel-Forschung*, 20 (7): 912–13.

Muthén, B. (1984) 'A general structural equation model with dichotomous, ordered categorical, and continuous latent variable indicators', *Psychometrika*, 49: 115–32.

National Institutes of Health (1972) *The Women and their Pregnancies*, DHEW publication (NIH) 73–379. Washington, DC: US Government Printing Office.

Pearl, J. (1988) *Probabilistic Reasoning in Intelligent Systems: Networks of Plausible Inference*. San Mateo, CA: Morgan Kaufmann.

Schmitt, N. (1990) 'Stadieneinteilung chronischer Schmerzen'. Medical dissertation, University of Mainz.

Simpson, E.H. (1951) 'The interpretation of interaction in contingency tables', *Journal of the Royal Statistical Society, Series B*, 13: 238–41.

Spielberger, C.D. (1983) *Manual for the State-Trait Anxiety Inventory*. Palo Alto: Consulting Psychologists Press.

Wermuth, N. (1989) 'Parametric collapsibility and the lack of moderating effects in contingency tables with a dichotomous response variable', *Journal of the Royal Statistical Society, Series B*, 49: 353–64.

Wermuth, N. (1992a) 'On moderating effects in the interactional and in the confounding sense, a reply', *Methodika*, 6: 5–7.

Wermuth, N. (1992b) 'On block-recursive regression equations (with discussion)', *Brazilian Journal of Probability and Statistics*, 6: 1–56.

Wermuth, N. and Cox, D.R. (1992a) 'Derived variables calculated from similar responses: some characteristics and examples', *Computational Statistics and Data Analysis*.

Wermuth, N. and Cox, D.R. (1992b) 'On the relations between interactions obtained with alternative codings of discrete variables', *Methodika*, 6: 76–85.

Wermuth, N. and Cox, D.R. (1992c) 'Graphical models for dependencies and associations' in Y. Dodge and J. Whittaker (eds), *Computational Statistics, vol. 1*. Heidelberg: Physica, pp. 235–49.

Wermuth, N. and Koller, S. (1976) 'Systematik multivariater Korrelationsmuster angewandt auf die Symptomkorrelation von Krankheiten', in S. Koller and J. Berger (eds), *Klinisch-Statistische Forschung*. Stuttgart: Schattauer. pp. 111–20.

Wermuth, N. and Lauritzen, S.L. (1983) 'Graphical and recursive models for contingency tables', *Biometrika*, 70: 537–52.

Wermuth, N. and Lauritzen, S.L. (1990) 'On substantive research hypotheses, conditional independence graphs and graphical chain models (with discussion)', *Journal of the Royal Statistical Society, Series B*, 52: 21–72.

Wold, H.O. (1954) 'Causality and econometrics', *Econometrica*, 22: 162–77.

10

Specification and Estimation of Latent Variable Models

Gerhard Arminger

Basic Ideas of Latent Variable Models

In this chapter, concepts for the construction and estimation of statistical models with latent variables are presented. The literature on this subject is vast, and hence only selected topics that are deemed to be especially important for population health research are covered here. Before latent variable models are introduced in a more formal way, some basic distinctions to classify latent variable models are discussed.

Platonic and Operational Variables

In general we think of a latent variable, denoted by η, as a random variable whose outcome cannot be observed directly but is a variable of genuine substantive interest for the researcher. The first distinction we have to make is whether a variable can be observed directly – at least in principle – or whether it can never be observed directly. In the first case η is called a platonic variable, and an observed variable y may be a good or bad approximation of it, but in any case the true relation between η and y may be obtained from elements of a population in which both η and y are directly observed. A typical example for a platonic variable is the blood pressure η of a person during a given period, which at least in principle may be measured correctly through direct observation, while the answer to the question of whether the person experienced symptoms of hypertension could be used as an approximation y.

The second type of variable is called an operational variable, in which the relationship between η and y is always given by some model and cannot be obtained from population elements where both η and y can be observed. The substantive meaning of η is then defined by the observed variable y and the selected model and is not an inherent characteristic of y. In this case, not all but maybe only a few consequences of a proposed model for the relation between y

and η can be tested with empirical data. Conclusions drawn from such operational variables are of course much weaker than from platonic variables. Typical examples for operational variables are 'intelligence' measured as the score of some intelligence tests, or 'lifestyle' indirectly observed through questions on consumer behaviour. Unfortunately, operational variables are often encountered in epidemiology when the effects of vaguely defined but possibly important variables such as dietary habits and lifestyle on health risks are studied. Although operational variables may be constructed 'theoretically' – such a construct is 'paranoia' in psychiatry – all variables that cannot be measured directly at all, that is all variables that are not platonic, cause great problems of interpretation which are discussed in detail in Bielby (1986) and Sobel and Arminger (1986).

Single-Indicator Models
The second distinction is between single- and multiple-indicator models. The reasons for developing single- and multiple-indicator models are quite different. In the first case the latent variable η is observed through only one variable y. Single-indicator models typically occur when the measurement level of η and the measurement level of the observed variable y are different. While η is usually a metric variable, y may be censored metric, dichotomous, ordered or unordered categorical. In applications we are often interested in estimating the influence of some explanatory variables $x_1, \ldots, x_p$ on η, but only y has been observed. The relation between y, η and x may be represented as in Figure 10.1. Only the

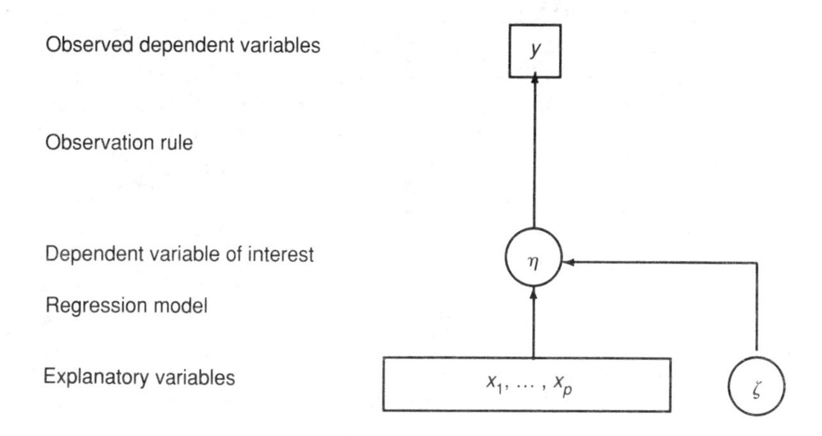

Figure 10.1 *A regression model for a latent variable*

variables y and $x_1, \ldots, x_p$ can be observed; the variable η and the error ζ are unobserved.

A typical example is a simple model to formulate the dependency of colon cancer on meat intake x_1 and potato intake x_2. We can think of a latent variable η which is regarded as the disposition to develop colon cancer. A regression equation for η with ζ is given by

$$\eta = \beta_0 + x_1\beta_1 + x_2\beta_2 + \zeta$$

However, η cannot be observed directly. A rather crude measurement of η is given by the following observation rule:

$$y = \begin{cases} 0 & \text{if } \eta \leq \tau \text{ (no cancer)} \\ 1 & \text{if } \eta > \tau \text{ (cancer)} \end{cases}$$

The threshold τ is the critical value which must be crossed to develop colon cancer. In this example one observes a single dichotomous indicator of a latent variable η. If ζ is assumed to be standard normal and τ is set to 0 for identification, the parameters β_0, β_1 and β_2 may be estimated from a sample $\{y_i, x_{i1}, x_{i2}\}$, $i = 1, \ldots, n$ of independent observations using a binomial probit model. The observation rule connects the latent variable η and the observed variable y. The most important examples are the following:

1 The identity relation in which y and η are metric:

$$y = \eta$$

2 The factor analytic model in which y and η are metric:

$$y = \alpha + \lambda\eta + \epsilon$$

This model is a simple extension of the identity relation. The variable of interest η is disturbed by a measurement error ϵ, a scale factor λ and a shift variable α which may cause an upward or downward bias.

3 The threshold model for a metric censored variable y with a known threshold τ and a metric latent variable η:

$$y = \begin{cases} \eta & \text{if } \eta > \tau \\ \tau & \text{if } \eta \leq \tau \end{cases}$$

4 The threshold model for an ordered categorical variable y and a metric latent variable η with unknown thresholds τ_k, $k = 0, \ldots, K$:

$$y = k \Longleftrightarrow \tau_{k-1} < \eta \leq \tau_k$$

The observed variable y takes on the value k if η falls between τ_{k-1} and τ_k. The value of τ_0 is set to $-\infty$, $\tau_k = +\infty$. The estimation of the thresholds depends on the distribution of η. Typically, the assumption of a normal distribution is made. This threshold model is probably the most useful model for sciences that work with ratings and judgements of individuals.

Multiple-Indicator Models

Multiple-indicator models were originally developed to measure unobserved variables such as intelligence with many indicators. The underlying assumption is that a score constructed from many measurements is more reliable and hopefully more valid than a simple approximation. Furthermore, one hopes that the use of many indicators can operationalize difficult theoretical concepts which cannot be observed directly. In a multiple-indicator model one or more latent variables η_j, $j = 1, \ldots, q$ are measured by indicators y_i, $i = 1, \ldots, p$. A simple example is a one-factor model

$$\begin{aligned} y_1 &= \alpha_1 + \lambda_1\eta + \epsilon_1 \\ y_2 &= \alpha_2 + \lambda_2\eta + \epsilon_2 \\ &\vdots \\ y_p &= \alpha_p + \lambda_p\eta + \epsilon_p \end{aligned}$$

in which one latent variable η is measured by p metric indicators. The measurement model takes the form of a linear multivariate regression of $y \sim p \times 1$ on η with regression constants α_i, regression coefficients λ_i and errors ϵ_i. In this context α_i may be interpreted as bias of the indicator y_i, λ_i is called the loading of y_i on η and ϵ_i is interpreted as measurement error. If η and ϵ are uncorrelated, the variance $V(y_i)$ of y_i is decomposed into

$$V(y_i) = \lambda_i^2 V(\eta) + V(\epsilon_i)$$

The proportion $\lambda_i^2 V(\eta)/V(y_i)$ may be interpreted as a coefficient of reliability of y_i as a measurement of η. This model is often appropriate if a variable such as intake of the amount of a certain kind of food is measured not only on one but on many occasions, or if physical activity is measured as time spent in different kinds of sports. A natural generalization of the single-factor model is the multiple-factor model when the observed variables y_i, $i = 1, \ldots, p$ load on several factors η_j, $j = 1, \ldots, q$. The corresponding measurement model is written in matrix notation as

$$y = \alpha + \Lambda\eta + \epsilon$$

with the constant vector $\alpha \sim p \times 1$, the loading matrix $\Lambda \sim p \times q$ and the error vector $\epsilon \sim q \times 1$, which is assumed to be uncorrelated with η. The covariance matrix Σ of y may then be decomposed into

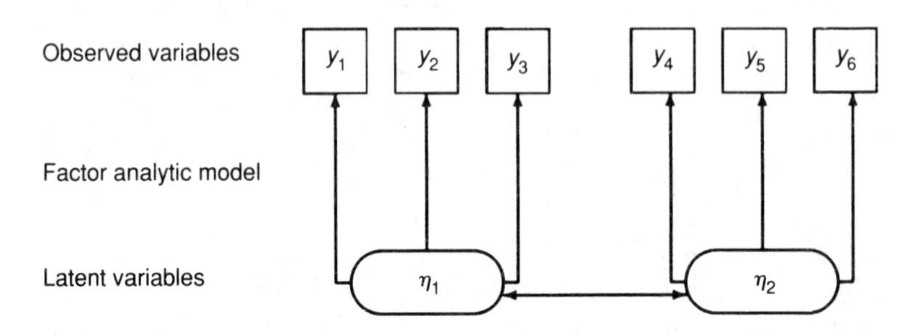

Figure 10.2 *A factor analytic measurement model*

$$\Sigma = \Lambda\Phi\Lambda^{T} + \Theta$$

where Φ is the covariance matrix of η and Θ is the covariance matrix of ϵ. A graphical representation of a factor analytic model with metric observed variables y_i and latent metric variables is given in Figure 10.2. Note that in a factor analytic model all of the indicators have a metric measurement level, which is a rather restrictive assumption.

Latent Traits and Latent Classes

The final distinction concerns the measurement level of a latent variable. If the latent variable is continuous, as is usually assumed for variables such as 'intelligence', 'physical activity' and 'food intake', the multiple-indicator models for η are often called latent trait models. If the variable η is unordered categorical with a finite number of L categories, the corresponding models are usually called latent class models. In this case interest usually focuses on the estimation of the probability that an individual falls into class l, that is $Pr(\eta = l) = \pi_l$. The latent class concept is useful in epidemiology if a set of symptoms $y_1, \ldots, y_p$ is used to determine whether somebody suffers from a certain type of illness ($\eta = 1$) or not ($\eta = 2$) (see Eaton and Bohrnstedt, 1989). The latent class model for unordered categorical y_i with categories $k = 1, \ldots, K$ and unordered categorical η with categories $l = 1, \ldots, L$ is given by

$$Pr(y_i = k) = \sum_{l=1}^{L} Pr(y_i = k|\eta = l)Pr(\eta = l)$$

Note that for metric as well as for categorical latent variables, η may depend on a vector x. In fact, this dependency may be of central interest for the substantive researcher.

A General Conceptual Framework for Latent Variable Models

Combining Regression and Indicator Models

In practical research, all of the categories of the distinctions that have been made above may be combined in almost any way. A realistic model in epidemiology may contain metric dependent latent variables such as dieting habits which are measured by metric, dichotomous and/or ordered categorical variables. The dieting habits may in turn influence certain risk factors which are again measured by multiple indicators. The dieting habits may depend on physical activity and socio-economic variables which may have to be observed indirectly through indicators of different measurement levels. The idea is to combine the different elements of the distinctions made in the first section of this chapter to define a model that is tailored to the needs of the substantive researcher. One usually starts with the definition of the joint dependent variables in a model. A variable is always a dependent variable if it cannot be observed directly, that is if it is a latent variable and/or if it depends on other dependent variables or on explanatory variables. The explanatory variables, which may be metric or dummy variables, are collected in a vector x. The latent dependent variables are collected in a vector η. The latent variables η and the explanatory variables x are connected through a regression or a simultaneous equation model. If there are multiple indicators for the vector η, a factor analytic model is used to connect η with the indicators. If the indicators are all metric then they are observed directly and are denoted by the vector y. However, it may be necessary to introduce additional latent variables denoted by y^* if the measurement level of the observed variables is non-metric. In this case a factor analytic model connects the latent variables η and the latent indicators y^*, while the latent variables y^* are linked to the observed variables y through an observation rule. The graphical representation of such a general model is found in Küsters and Schepers (1990). The following notation is used:

y_{11} metric indicator connected with metric y^*_{11} through the identity relation

y_{12} censored metric indicator connected with metric y^*_{12} through a threshold model

y_{13} ordered categorical indicator connected with metric y^*_{13} through a threshold model

y_{21} ordered categorical indicator connected with metric y^*_{21} through a threshold model

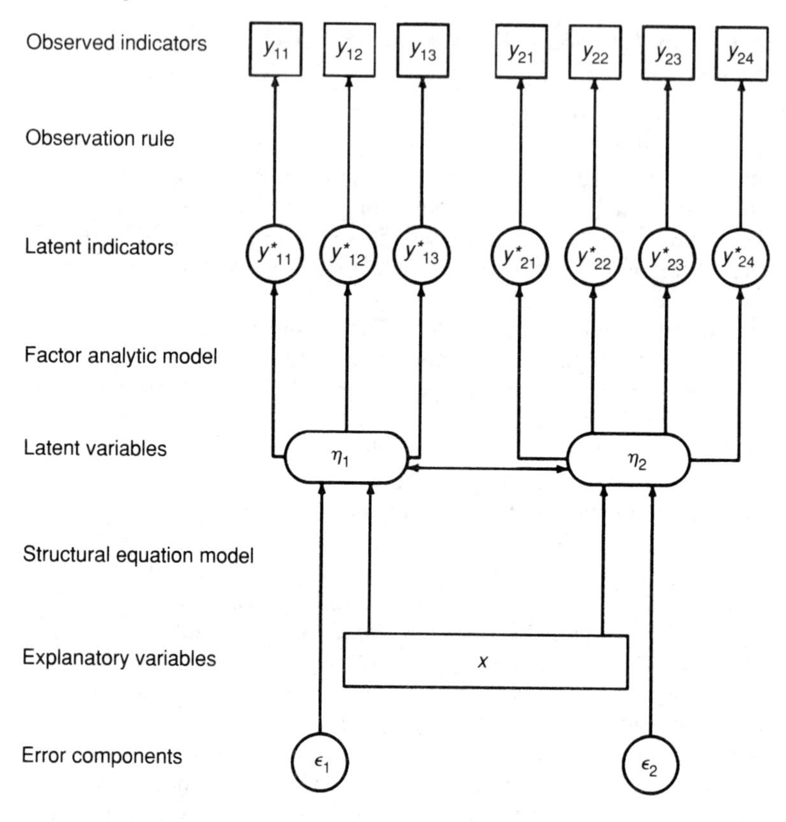

Figure 10.3 *Combined regression and measurement models in latent variables with metric and non-metric indicators*

- y_{22} metric indicator (a count variable) connected with metric y^*_{22} through a log-linear model
- y_{23} unordered categorical indicator connected with metric y^*_{23} through a multinomial logit model
- y_{24} metric indicator connected with metric y^*_{24} through the identity relation.

Figure 10.3 represents a conceptually unified treatment of regression models with multiple indicators that may have metric and/or non-metric measurement levels. However, the conceptual model is only the first step to specify and to estimate the relations that link x and y. The second step is the formulation of a corresponding probability model.

Mixture Distributions

In this section some of the construction principles for latent variable models of Arminger and Küsters (1989) are used, which are based on the original formulation of latent structure models by Lazarsfeld and Henry (1968). In general the random vectors y, η and x are considered where the components of y and x are observed in sampling units while η is fully missing. The components of each vector may be of any measurement level. The marginal density function of each component will be either a discrete probability or a continuous density function or a mixed discrete/continuous density. The joint density will also be a mixed discrete/continous density function. Let $P(x)$ denote the marginal density of x, $P(\eta|x)$ the conditional density of η given x and $P(y|\eta, x)$ the conditional density of y given η and x. The conditional density $P(y|x)$ of y given x is given by the mixture density

$$P(y|x) = \int_{D(\eta)} P(y|\eta, x)P(\eta|x)d\eta$$

where $D(\eta)$ denotes the domain of η and the integration is taken over the components of η. Note that this is only a more complicated way of writing the theorem of complete probability

$$P(A) = \sum_{k=1}^{k} P(A|E_k)P(E_k)$$

where A is any event and E_k, $k = 1, \ldots, K$ is a partition of the event space Ω. The mixture density equation is only a simple identity but it allows the researcher to decompose the density $P(y|x)$ into a mixing density $P(\eta|x)$ that models the dependence of the latent variables on the explanatory variables x and a conditional density that models the dependence of y on η and x. $P(\eta|x)$ may be considered as a reduced form model that gives the total effects of x on η from which the structural form may be deduced if identifiability conditions are met. Usually the researcher will be most interested in the structural form. The conditional density $P(y|\eta, x)$ may be considered as a measurement model that allows the researcher to make some inferences about the kind and the quality of the measurements used in the study. To obtain a useful model, restrictions have to be put on the mixing as well as on the conditional density.

Specification of the Mixing Density The latent variable vector η usually consists only of continuous variables (latent trait models) or only of unordered categorical variables (latent class models). If η

consists of more than one unordered categorical variable then the combinations of these categorical variables may be written as the cells of a multidimensional contingency table. Such a table can always be written as one unordered categorical variable where the number of categories is equal to the number of possible combinations of the categories of the original variable. Hence in latent class models one usually considers only the case of one categorical variable. The mixing density is then given by

$$P(\eta|x) = P(\eta = l|x), \quad l = 1, \ldots, L$$

In latent class models η very often does not depend on x. Exceptions are found in Clogg and Goodman (1984) where x indexes multiple groups and $P(\eta = l)$ varies over the different groups, and in Formann (1985) where restrictions across the probabilities of belonging to a class $l = 1, \ldots, L$ are parameterized with a design matrix. In general, dependence of η on x can easily be incorporated into a latent class model by using one of the conventional regression models for dependent categorical variables such as the multinomial logit model. However, at least to my knowledge, general dependencies of η on x have not been included in computer programs that estimate latent class models.

While latent class models usually consider only one latent variable that does not depend on some x, latent trait models are often formulated as structural equation systems in which a vector of continuous dependent variables is dependent on itself as well as on some explanatory variables x. A special case of such a structural equation system is the path models used in sociological research. In the context of mixing densities such a model is considered as a special case of $P(\eta|x)$ in which the expected value of η given x is a linear model in x and additional assumptions are made about the covariance matrix and possibly about the joint distribution of the disturbance terms ζ. Let $\eta \sim q \times 1$ be a vector of endogenous variables, and $x \sim n \times 1$ be a vector of exogenous variables including a regression constant, which are related to each other in the structural equation model

$$\eta = B\eta + \Gamma x + \zeta$$

where the disturbance ζ has expected value 0 and a covariance matrix Ψ. The errors are assumed to be independent of x and $(I - B)$ is a non-singular matrix. Important special cases are univariate and multivariate regression ($B = 0$) and the recursive or path analytic models where B is lower triangular. If the indicators of the latent variables are continuous it is not necessary to specify the density $P(\eta|x)$ for the estimation of B,Γ and Ψ further, as will be explained later. However, in the general case with non-metric variables as indicators it will be necessary to specify the density $P(\eta|x)$ fully. In this case, multivariate normality of ζ is assumed throughout the chapter so that $\zeta \sim \mathcal{N}(0,\Psi)$. Of course this specification of the mixing density is not the only useful and sensible specification but it is certainly the most common one and is familiar to researchers working with regression and analysis of variance models. It is assumed that the model is first- and second-order identified, that is if the parameters of B, Γ and Ψ are collected in a vector ϑ and the vectors ϑ_1 and ϑ_2 yield the same mean and covariance matrix of η for given x then ϑ_1 and ϑ_2 must be equal.

Specification of the Conditional Density Note that the specification of the conditional density $P(y|\eta, x)$ of y given (η, x) in the mixture equation is independent of the model for (η, x). Hence, continuous as well as discrete values for η may be used. Before we turn to distributional assumptions about $P(y|\eta, x)$ we consider three important simplifications of $P(y|\eta, x)$ which are often made to construct models that are substantively meaningful, have identifiable parameter structures and can be estimated with the usual estimation principles and the tools of modern statistical computing.

The first simplification eliminates the dependence of y on x by replacing $P(y|\eta, x)$ through $P(y|\eta)$, where y depends on x only through η and no longer directly on x. Substantively, this replacement makes sense if the measurement of η through y does not depend on the regressor variables x. Of course, this simplification cannot be used if the measurement part of the model is different for the regressors in x. A typical example for different measurement structures is in psychological tests when it is believed that men and women respond differently to a set of items, which may imply different patterns and loadings in the factor loading matrix for a factor analysis of the item set. In such a case, x may index multiple groups, that is the population consists of heterogeneous subpopulations. Consequently, some programs like LISREL and LISCOMP provide multiple-group options for latent trait models, and Clogg and Goodman (1984) deal with latent class analysis in multiple groups. In the rest of this chapter only the simplified conditional density $P(y|\eta)$ is considered.

The second simplification is not of theoretical but of great practical importance for the estimation of models with ordered or unordered categorical indicators for latent traits. If one assumes that the vector y of indicators can be partitioned in such a way that each component y_i loads on only one latent variable η_j, then the estimation can be simplified greatly. This simplification is a special form of Thurstone's (1947) simple structure. Substantively, it means that the items in a subset of items lie on one dimension of the factor space and that all items that lie on more than one factor have been eliminated from this particular subset. This assumption usually makes it much easier for the researcher to identify a latent trait substantively and to interpret factor loadings and regression coefficients in the simultaneous equation model.

The third simplification is the assumption of local independence between the indicator variables given η

$$P(y|\eta) = \prod_{i=1}^{p} P(y_i|\eta)$$

Substantively, it implies that the statistical association between the indicators y_i is generated only by their common dependence on η. If η is held constant, then this association disappears and the indicators are statistically independent. While this notion has certainly been dominant in shaping the thinking of psychometricians and statisticians about latent variable models and factor analysis (see for instance Bartholomew, 1987), I do not believe that it is an absolutely necessary concept for latent variable models. As an important exception, consider the case of a panel or cohort study in which the same questions are asked from the same individuals at successive times. In this case, the error terms in the measurement model will be serially correlated if metric indicators are used and the local independence assumption is not appropriate (Corballis and Traub, 1970).

We turn now to typical examples for the specification of the conditional density $P(y|\eta)$:

1 The factor analytic model for metric y and continuous η is given by

$$y = \Lambda\eta = \epsilon$$

in which $\Lambda \sim p \times q$ is the loading matrix, $E(\epsilon) = 0, V(\epsilon) = \Theta$ and ϵ is assumed to be independent of η. If the second simplification holds, then Λ has a simple structure of the block diagonal form:

$$\Lambda = \begin{bmatrix} \Lambda_1 & 0 & \dots & 0 \\ 0 & \Lambda_2 & \dots & 0 \\ \vdots & \vdots & \ddots & \vdots \\ 0 & 0 & \dots & \Lambda_q \end{bmatrix}$$

If the assumption of local independence holds, then Θ is a diagonal matrix. The diagonal elements θ_{ii} contain the variance of the measurement error which can be used as a measure of the reliability of the measurements. As in the structural equation model, the conditional density $P(y|\eta)$ is until now only specified in the first two moments. A full specification of $P(y|\eta)$ is achieved if $\epsilon \sim \mathcal{N}(0,\Theta)$.

2 The threshold model for censored y_i and a continuous vector η. Latent indicators y_i^* are introduced which are collected in the vector y^*. This vector y^* is modelled in the same factor analytic structure as y in the first example:

$$y^* = \Lambda\eta + \epsilon$$

The measurement error ϵ is assumed to be normal. If the threshold model

$$y_i = \begin{cases} y_i^* & \text{if } y_i^* > \tau_i \\ \tau_i^* & \text{if } y_i^* \leq \tau_i \end{cases}$$

with known threshold τ_i is tagged on to the factor analytic structure for y_i^*, then the univariate conditional density function is the univariate normal density if $y_i^* > \tau_i$. Otherwise the univariate conditional probability, that is $P(y_i = \tau_i|x_i)$, is the integrated normal density with lower bound $-\infty$ and upper bound τ_i if $y_i^* \leq \tau_i$. This is the Tobit regression model for censored dependent variables (Tobin, 1958; Amemiya, 1984). In contrast to the factor analytic model, the full distributional specification of $P(y_i|\eta)$ is essential for estimation.

3 Very similar to the Tobit model for censored variables is the ordinal probit model (McKelvey and Zavoina, 1975) for an ordered categorical variable y_i with unknown thresholds τ_i, and K_i categories. The factor analytic structure of y^* is the same as in the second example. Additionally the threshold model

$$y_i = k \Longleftrightarrow \tau_{\text{i},k-1} < y_i^* \leq \tau_{i,K_i}$$

is tagged on. The univariate conditional density $\text{P}(y_i = k|\eta)$ is then given by the integrated normal density between $\tau_{i,k-1}$ and τ_{i,k_i} with $\tau_{i,0}$ and $= -\infty$ and $\tau_{i,K_i} = +\infty$. In the case of the ordinal probit, additional restrictions must be introduced to identify the loading parameters $\lambda_{i,j}$. If η contains a constant as one of its components, the corresponding regression constant or one of the thresholds must be set to a constant. Usually $\tau_{i,1}$ is set to 0. Since the ordered categorical variable y_i has no natural scale, the variance of ϵ_i is set to 1 (see Nelson, 1976). In contrast to the Tobit model, the thresholds $\tau_{i,k}$ are estimated from the data. Again, the full distributional specification of $P(y_i|\eta)$ is necessary for estimation.

4 The latent class model for unordered categorical variables y_i and one unordered categorical variable η with L categories. In latent

class models usually all of the indicators are assumed to be unordered categorical with K_i categories and the assumption of local independence is invoked. Hence the conditional density $P(y|\eta)$ is given by

$$P(y|\eta) = \Pr(y_1 = k_1, \ldots, y_p = k_p|\eta = l) = \prod_{i=1}^{p} P(y_i = k_i|\eta = l)$$

The univariate conditional probabilities $P(y_i = k_i|\eta = l)$ are to be estimated. A model for unordered categorical indicators with latent traits η is difficult to formulate. Hence the reader is referred to Arminger and Küsters (1989).

Some Common Latent Variable Models

In this section the specifications of the mixing density and the conditional density given in the previous sections are combined to generate some common latent variable models. The focus is on model generation, but some remarks regarding the estimation of the parameters and computer programs are given. Only models that can be estimated with publicly available computer programs are considered in detail.

The Latent Class Model

The latent class models (Lazarsfeld and Henry, 1968; Goodman, 1974; McCutcheon, 1987; Langeheine, 1988) usually consider p unordered categorical variables y_i with K_i categories as indicators of a latent variable with L categories which is not dependent on explanatory variables x. Under the assumption of local independence, the joint distribution of the vector y is given by

$$P(y) = \Pr(y_1 = k_1, \ldots, y_p = k_p) = \sum_{l=1}^{L} \prod_{i=1}^{p} P(y_i = k_i|\eta = l)P(\eta = l)$$

The parameters that are to be estimated are the conditional univariate probabilities $P(y_i = k_i|\eta = l)$ and the mixing probabilities $P(\eta = l)$. If the variables y_i are symptoms of an illness then η is considered to be the dichotomous variable indicating that somebody is sick ($\eta = 1$) or not ($\eta = 2$). The mixing probability $P(\eta = 1)$ can then be considered as the prevalence of the illness and the conditional probabilities tell us how likely it is that a positive symptom occurs if somebody is sick or not. If the researcher is interested in the probability that somebody is sick, given a symptom is positive, he has to compute the posterior Bayes probability $P(\eta = 1|y_i = 1)$ which can be deduced from the last equation.

The mixing and conditional probabilities are conventionally estimated with maximum likelihood methods from a random sample of size N using a multinomial model for a p-dimensional contingency table. If h denotes the cell combination $\{k_1, \ldots, k_p\}$, π_h the probability under the model, f_h the absolute frequency of this combination and H the number of combinations that have been observed, then the log-likelihood function is given by

$$l(\vartheta) = \sum_{h=1}^{H} f_h \log \pi_h(\vartheta)$$

where ϑ is the $t \times 1$ parameter vector to be estimated consisting of the mixing and the conditional probabilities. If the model is correctly specified, the likelihood ratio test statistic or the corresponding χ^2 statistic is asymptotically χ^2 distributed with $H - t$ degrees of freedom. The estimated parameters are consistent and asymptotically normal. The asymptotic covariance matrix of the parameters is estimated from inverting the matrix of second derivatives of the log-likelihood function which consistently estimates the Fisher information matrix.

The log-likelihood function that must be maximized in ϑ looks deceptively simple. However, it must be kept in mind that the basis of information is the p-dimensional contingency table of the observed variables, which at least for large p often has more cells than sample elements. As an example, consider ten dichotomous variables as indicators for a latent class variable. To find reliable parameter estimates the probabilities of the corresponding contingency table with 1024 cells have to be estimated from the sample. As a consequence, only fairly small models have been estimated in actual research, as illustrated by the analysis of the data of a large study of approximately 3000 psychiatric patients performed by specialists in latent class methodology (Eaton and Bohrnstedt, 1989).

Clogg and Goodman (1984) have extended latent class analysis to the multiple-group case. Langeheine (1988) considers the analysis of latent classes over time, and Rost (1988) has extended latent class methodology to ordered categorical indicators. A treatment of latent class models for measuring, including the relation of these models to latent trait models with dichotomous indicators introduced by Rasch (1980), is found in Clogg (1988).

Mean and Covariance Structure Models

Mean and covariance structure models comprise a large class of models for metric indicators y of continous latent variables η that may depend on continuous and/or categorical regressors x. These models have become very popular through accessible computer programs like LISREL 7 (Jöreskog and Sörbom, 1988) and EQS (Bentler, 1985). To construct a mean and covariance structure model, the mixing density of a simultaneous equation system under the assumption of multivariate normality of ζ (as given earlier) is combined with the conditional density of a factor analytic model (also given earlier). Again, multivariate normality of the error term ϵ is assumed. Then y given x follows the conditional normal density:

$$y \sim \mathcal{N}(\Lambda\Pi x, \Lambda\Omega\Lambda^{T} + \Theta)$$

Here Π is the matrix of reduced form regression coefficients, given by

$$\Pi = (I - B)^{-1}\Gamma$$

The parameters of the model are collected in a parameter vector $\vartheta \sim t \times 1$ which is estimated from a random sample of size N.

The usual estimation procedure to estimate ϑ is the maximum likelihood estimation method in which the log-likelihood function

$$l(\vartheta) = \sum_{h=1}^{N} log\ \varphi(y_h|\Lambda\Pi x_h, \Lambda\Omega\Lambda' + \Theta)$$

of the sample is maximized as a function of ϑ. $\varphi(.|.,.)$ is the multivariate normal density with expected value $\Lambda\Pi x_h$ and covariance matrix $\Lambda\Omega\Lambda^{T} + \Theta$. The estimated parameters are consistent and asymptotically normal; the asymptotic covariance matrix of the parameters is estimated from inverting the matrix of second derivatives of the log-likelihood function which consistently estimates the Fisher information matrix. A necessary requirement for correct specification is the first- and second-order identifiability of the specified model defined in the same way as for the simultaneous equation system given earlier. Because the model is highly non-linear in the parameters, no identification rules can be given for the general model. Only the local identification status can be checked by computing the rank of the Fisher information matrix at the parameter estimate $\hat{\vartheta}$ (McDonald and Krane, 1977).

There has been a protracted discussion about possible consequences of non-normality of y given x in such models. To avoid possible negative consequences Browne (1984) has developed the asymptotically distribution-free (ADF) estimator. For the computation of the ADF estimator the empirical variances and covariances of y and x are collected in a vector s_N; the corresponding elements of the covariance matrices under the model parameterized in ϑ are collected in a vector $\sigma(\vartheta)$. Then the Mahalanobis distance

$$Q(\vartheta) = (s_N - \sigma(\vartheta))'\hat{W}^{-1}(s - \sigma(\vartheta))$$

between the two vectors is minimized. If the weight matrix $(1/N)\hat{W}$ is a consistent estimator of the asymptotic covariance matrix of $(\sqrt{N})s_N$, then the estimated parameters are consistent and asymptotically normal although multivariate normality of y given x has not been assumed. However, since $\hat{W}$ is an empirical covariance matrix of a covariance matrix, the elements of $\hat{W}$ have to be computed from the empirical moments of the fourth order, which is very time consuming. Additionally, the number of parameters that must be estimated from the sample grows very rapidly with the number of variables in the model. Consider a simple factor analytic model with $p = 15$ variables. The number of elements in s_N *is 120, the number of elements in* $\hat{W}$ that have to be computed from the sample is 7260, and the 120×120 matrix has to be inverted in the minimization procedure. Hence, the ADF method is stable only for fairly large samples of size $N = 1000$ or more.

A different approach to deal with the consequences of nonnormality that avoids the computational difficulties of ADF estimation has been proposed by Arminger and Schoenberg (1989) based on the theory of pseudo maximum likelihood (PML) estimation developed by Gourieroux et al. (1984). First, it is shown that the maximum likelihood (ML) estimator always yields consistent parameter estimates regardless of the distribution of y given x if first- and second-order identifiability holds. Secondly, it is shown that, in general, the ML estimator of the asymptotic covariance matrix of the ML parameter estimates is inconsistent. However, a consistent estimator of this covariance matrix can be computed if the first and second derivatives of the log-likelihood function are used and not just the first or the second derivatives as in ML estimation. PML estimation of mean and covariance structure models has been implemented in the program LINCS (Schoenberg, 1989) and will be implemented in the procedure CALIS of the SAS system.

The mean and covariance structures presented here have been generalized in three ways. First, if x indexes heterogeneous subpopulations then the measurement model $P(y|\eta, x)$ may be specific for each group, and multiple-group models have to be estimated and restrictions across groups may have to be imposed (see Jöreskog and Sörbom, 1988). Secondly, the number of levels in which latent variables occur have been extended from one to many by McDonald (1978; 1980). Thirdly, the random coefficient models of regression analysis and analysis of variance have recently been extended to factor analysis and mean and covariance structure models by Muthén (1989). Note that all of these models can be formulated as mean and covariance structure models in which means $\mu(x;\vartheta,g)$ and covariance matrices $\Sigma(\vartheta,g)$ of the observed variables y given x are structured as functions of ϑ for heterogeneous populations $g = 1, \ldots, G$.

Mean and Covariance Structure Models with Non-Metric Dependent Variables

While the mean and covariance structure models formulated in the previous section are already fairly general, they are not necessarily well suited to research in epidemiology and social medicine, where many of the observed variables are not continuous but are censored on one or on both sides, are classified metric, or are dichotomous or ordered categorical. If one is willing to assume that these observed variables y_i are generated from unobserved variables y_i^* through the threshold models discussed earlier, then the mean and covariance structures of the previous section can be expanded to include such non-metric dependent variables on the condition that the disturbances ζ_j of the simultaneous equation model and the errors ϵ_i of the measurement model are jointly normal given x. Such models have been constructed and estimated by Muthén (1984); the consistency and asymptotic normality of the estimators proposed by Muthén have been proved by Küsters (1987).

The construction of these models closely follows Figure 10.3. First, the mean and covariance structure model is formulated in the variables y_i^*, $i = 1, \ldots, p$ yielding the mixture density

$$P(y^*|x) = \varphi(y^*|\Lambda\Pi x, \Lambda\Omega\Lambda' + \Theta)$$

Secondly, each variable y_i^* is linked to the corresponding component y_i by a threshold model with a normal error. The thresholds are known if y_i is censored or classified metric; they are not known if y_i is ordered categorical. If x in the last equation includes a constant term as its first component, an identification restriction like $\tau_{i,1} = 0$ must be imposed. As discussed before, the variance of y_i^* must be restricted to a constant (such as 1). Otherwise the threshold model will not be identified (Nelson, 1976). If one considers the scalar variable y_i given x, the univariate marginal density $P(y_i|x)$ is either a univariate normal density or a probability defined by the normal cumulative distribution function integrating over y_i^* within the boundaries $\tau_{i,k-1}$ and $\tau_{i,k}$. If one looks at the variables y_i and y_j given x, their joint marginal density is given either by a bivariate normal density or by the integration over y_i^* and/or y_j^* in a bivariate normal density within the boundaries $\tau_{i,k-1}$ and $\tau_{i,k}$ and/or $\tau_{j,l-1}$ and $\tau_{j,l}$.

The normal distribution is completely characterized if the means and the variances of each variable y_i^* and the covariances between each pair of variables y_i^* and y_j^* given x are known. Hence, Muthén

(1984) bases his estimation procedure completely on the densities and probabilities obtained from the one- and two-dimensional normal densities. Let $\vartheta \sim t \times 1$ be the parameter vector of all threshold parameters τ, regression coefficients B and Γ, loadings Λ and covariance matrices Ω and Θ that have to be estimated from a random sample of size N. Let $M = \Lambda\Pi$ and $\Sigma = \Lambda\Omega\Lambda' + \Theta$. Then the estimation of ϑ is done in three stages (see Schepers et al., 1990).

In the first stage the threshold parameters τ, the reduced form coefficients M of the regression equation, and the reduced form error variances σ_i^2, $i = 1, \ldots, p$ are estimated using marginal maximum likelihood. The regression constant is the first component of the ith row of $M_{i\cdot}$ of M. The parameters to be estimated in the equation for variable y_i are the thresholds denoted by the vector τ_i, the regression coefficients, that is the ith row of M, and the variance denoted by σ_i^2. The log-likelihood function that is maximized with respect to $\{\tau_i, M_{i\cdot}, \sigma_i^2\}$ is given by

$$l_i(\tau_i, M_{i\cdot}, \sigma_i^2) = \sum_{h=1}^{N} \ln P(y_{hi}|x_h)$$

The formulation of $P(y_{hi}|x_h)$ depends on the measurement level of the observed variable y_i. If y_i is metric then $P(y_{hi}|x_h)$ is the univariate normal density with expected value $M_{i\cdot}x_h$ and variance σ_i^2. If y_i is an ordinal variable then the thresholds $\tau_{i,k}$ and the regression coefficients $M_{i\cdot}$ must be calculated from $P(y_{hi} = k|x_t)$ as in the ordinal probit model (McKelvey and Zavoina, 1975). If other models are used such as the Tobit model (Tobin, 1958) for dependent variables censored on one side only, the two-limit probit model (Rosett and Nelson, 1975) for dependent variables censored on both sides, or the model of Stewart (1983) for grouped metric variables, then the probabilities $P(y_{hi}|x_h)$ have to be modified accordingly.

A solution to the likelihood equations obtained by setting the first derivatives of $l_i(\tau_i, M_{i\cdot}, \sigma_i^2)$ to 0 is computed by applying a quasi-Newton algorithm. The second-order derivatives are approximated by computing the cross-product of the first-order derivatives. The first estimation stage yields strongly consistent estimates of $\tau_i, M_{i\cdot}$ and σ_i^2 for each equation i. Regularity conditions and the proof of strong consistency are given in Küsters (1987).

In the second stage the problem is to estimate the covariances of the error terms in the reduced form equations. Since the errors are assumed to be normally distributed, and strongly consistent estimators of the reduced form coefficients have already been obtained in the first stage, the estimation problem reduces to maximizing the log-likelihood function

$$l_{ij}(\sigma_{ij}) = \sum_{h=1}^{N} \ln P(y_{hi}, y_{hj}|x_h, \hat{\tau}_i, \hat{M}_{i\cdot}, \hat{\sigma}_i^2, \hat{\tau}_j, \hat{M}_{j\cdot}, \hat{\sigma}_j^2, \sigma_{ij})$$

in which $P(y_{hi}, y_{hj}|x_h, \hat{\tau}_i, \hat{M}_{i\cdot}, \hat{\sigma}_i^2, \hat{\tau}_j, \hat{M}_{j\cdot}, \hat{\sigma}_j^2, \sigma_{ij})$ is the bivariate probability of y_{hi} and y_{hj} given x_h and the reduced form coefficients. Note that in the ordinal case $\hat{\sigma}_i^2 = \hat{\sigma}_j^2 = 1$. Hence, σ_{ij} is a correlation coefficient which is called the polychoric correlation coefficient (Olsson, 1979). The log-likelihood function $l_{ij}(\sigma_{ij})$ has to be modified accordingly if variables with other measurement levels are used.

The objective function $l_{ij}(\sigma_{ij})$ is maximized using the *regula falsi* algorithm with analytical first derivatives. The resulting estimates $\hat{\sigma}_{ij}$ are strongly consistent estimators of σ_{ij}. Note that these covariances are the covariances of the error terms in the equations conditional on x_h. It is not assumed that the variables y^*_{hi} and y^*_{hj}, which depend on x_h, are normal; it is only assumed that the errors are normal.

The estimated thresholds $\hat{\tau}_i$, the reduced form coefficients $\hat{M}_{i\cdot}$, the variances $\hat{\sigma}_i^2$ and the covariances $\hat{\sigma}_{ij}$ from all equations are then collected in a vector $\hat{\kappa}_N$ which depends on the sample size N. For the final estimation stage, a strongly consistent estimate of the asymptotic covariance matrix W of $(\sqrt{N})\hat{\kappa}_N$ is computed. This estimate is denoted by $(1/N)\hat{W}_N$. The asymptotic covariance matrix W is difficult to derive since the estimates of the second stage depend on the estimated coefficients of the first stage. The various elements of the asymptotic covariance matrix W and a consistent estimator of W are found in Küsters (1987).

In the third stage the parameter vector ϑ is estimated by minimizing the Mahalanobis distance

$$Q_N(\vartheta) = (\hat{\kappa}_N - \kappa(\vartheta))'\hat{W}_N^{-1}(\hat{\kappa}_N - \kappa(\vartheta))$$

This procedure corresponds to a weighted least squares approach. The vector $(\sqrt{N})\hat{\kappa}_N$ is asymptotically normal with expected value $\kappa(\vartheta)$ and covariance matrix W. Since $(1/N)\hat{W}_N$ is a strongly consistent estimate of W, the quadratic form $Q_N(\vartheta)$ is centrally χ^2 distributed with $H - t$ degrees of freedom if the model is specified correctly and the sample size is sufficiently large. The number H indicates the number of elements in $\hat{\kappa}_N$. Note that this third stage is very similar to the estimation strategy employed for the ADF estimator in metric mean and covariance structure, so that the same remarks concerning the instability of the estimates due to insufficient sample size apply here too. In fact, because of the poor measurement level of many observed variables the sample size has to be even greater than in the metric case to obtain reliable parameter estimates.

The model specification and the estimation strategy presented here have been extended to the multiple-group case and have been implemented in three programs, LISREL 7 by Jöreskog and Sörbom (1988), LISCOMP by Muthén (1988) and MECOSA by Schepers and Arminger (1992). The disadvantage of LISREL 7 as compared with LISCOMP and MECOSA is that in LISREL 7 the parameter estimates of the first and second stage are not conditioned on x_h so that all variables y^* and x are assumed to be jointly multivariate normal. This assumption is unrealistic, since many explanatory variables are categorical and enter the simultaneous equation system as a vector of dummy variables. Note that, unlike in the metric mean and covariance structure estimation, there is no possibility of weakening the distributional assumptions given x. One pays for the low measurement level of the observed variables with stronger assumptions about the underlying density. The advantage of MECOSA over LISCOMP is that it allows the implementation of arbitrary restrictions on the parameters to be estimated. An example of such a non-linear restriction in a simultaneous probit model is found in Sobel and Arminger (1992).

Conclusion

In the previous section some important examples of latent variable models have been considered. Of course, there are many other possible combinations of mixing and conditional densities to generate latent variable models. A thorough discussion of factor analytic models for dichotomous and ordered categorical indicators without normality assumptions in the mixing density and alternative specifications of the conditional density are found in Bartholomew (1987). Arminger and Küsters (1989) have proposed and estimated a general latent trait model which allows indicators that are metric, censored metric, ordered categorical or unordered categorical under the assumption of simple structure and local independence. Here, the conditional density is not assumed to be normal. However, they have to use a two-stage marginal maximum likelihood estimator with a number of complications in the numerical algorithms which is different from the estimation approach outlined in the previous sections. The formulation and estimation of latent class models with explanatory variables x and indicators that are not unordered categorical apparently have not yet been considered in a general framework, although the use of metric, censored metric and ordered categorical indicators as symptoms for the presence or absence of a disease seem very natural.

Note

I wish to thank Kathryn Dean and Svend Kreiner for helpful comments on an earlier version of this paper and Bernd Weiler for his help in the preparation of the manuscript.

References

Amemiya, T. (1984) 'Tobit models: a survey', *Journal of Econometrics,* 24: 3–61.

Arminger, G. and Küsters, U. (1989) 'Construction principles for latent trait models', in C. C. Clogg (ed.), *Sociological Methodology 1989*. New York: Basil Blackwell. pp. 369–93.

Arminger, G. and Schoenberg, R. J. (1989) 'Pseudo maximum likelihood estimation and a test for misspecification in mean and covariance structure models', *Psychometrika,* 54: 409–25.

Bartholomew, D. J. (1987) *Latent Variable Models and Factor Analysis*. New York: Oxford University Press.

Bentler, P. M. (1985) *Theory and Implementation of EQS, a Structural Equations Program*. Los Angeles: BMDP Statistical Software.

Bielby, W. T. (1986) 'Arbitrary metrics in multiple indicator models of latent variables', *Sociological Methods and Research,* 15: 3–32.

Browne, M. W. (1984) 'Asymptotic distribution-free methods for the analysis of covariance structures', *British Journal of Mathematical Statistical Psychology,* 37: 62–83.

Clogg, C. C. (1988) 'Latent class models for measuring', in R. Langeheine and J. Rost (eds), *Latent Trait and Latent Class Models*. New York: Plenum. pp. 173–205.

Clogg, C. C. and Goodman, L. A. (1984) 'Latent structures analysis of a set of multidimensional contigency tables', *Journal of the American Statistical Association,* 79: 762–71.

Corballis, M. C. and Traub, R. E. (1970) 'Longitudinal factor analysis', *Psychometrika,* 35: 79–88.

Eaton, W. E. and Bohrnstedt, G. (eds) (1989) 'Latent variable models for dichotomous outcomes: analysis of data from the epidemiologic catchment area program', *Sociological Methods and Research, Special Issue*, 18 (1).

Formann, A. K. (1985) 'Constrained latent class models: theory and applications', *British Journal of Mathematical and Statistical Psychology,* 38: 87–111.

Goodman, L. A. (1974) 'Exploratory latent structure analysis using both identifiable and unidentifiable models', *Biometrika,* 61: 215–31.

Gourieroux, C., Monfort, A. and Trognon, A. (1984) 'Pseudo maximum likelihood methods: theory', *Econometrica,* 52: 681–700.

Jöreskog, K. G. and Sörbom, D. (1988) *LISREL 7 – A Guide to the Program and Applications*. Chicago: SPSS.

Küsters, U. (1987) *Hierarchische Mittelwert- und Kovarianzstrukturmodelle mit nichtmetrischen endogenen Variablen*, Heidelberg: Physica.

Küsters, U. and Schepers, A. (1990) 'Modelle zur Analyse von zensierten, dichotomen und ordinalen Paneldaten', in G. Arminger and F. Müller (eds), *Lineare*

Modelle zur Analyse von Paneldaten. Wiesbaden: Westdeutscher Verlag. pp. 173–202.

Langeheine, R. (1988) 'New developments in latent class theory', in R. Langeheine and J. Rost (eds), *Latent Trait and Latent Class Models*. New York: Plenum. pp. 77–108.

Lazarsfeld, P. F. and Henry, W. N. (1968) *Latent Structure Analysis*. Boston: Houghton Mifflin.

McCutcheon, A. (1987) *Latent Class Analysis*. Newbury Park, CA: Sage.

McDonald, R. P. (1978) 'A simple comprehensive model for the analysis of covariance structures', *British Journal of Mathematical and Statistical Psychology,* 31: 59–72.

McDonald, R. P. (1980) 'A simple comprehensive model for the analysis of covariance structures: some remarks on applications', *British Journal of Mathematical and Statistical Psychology,* 33: 161–83.

McDonald, R. P. and Krane, W. R. (1977) 'A note on local identifiability and degrees of freedom in the asymptotic likelihood ratio test', *British Journal of Mathematical and Statistical Psychology,* 30: 198–203.

McKelvey, R. D. and Zavoina, W. (1975) 'A statistical model for the analysis of ordinal level dependent variables', *Journal of Mathematical Sociology,* 4: 103–20.

Muthén, B. O. (1984) 'A general structural equation model with dichotomous, ordered categorical, and continuous latent variable indicators', *Psychometrika,* 49: 115–32.

Muthén, B. O. (1988) *LISCOMP – Analysis of Linear Equations Using a Comprehensive Measurement Model*. Mooresville: Scientific Software.

Muthén, B. O. (1989) 'Latent variable modeling in heterogeneous populations', *Psychometrika,* 54: 557–85.

Nelson, F. D. (1976) 'On a general computer algorithm for the analysis of models with limited dependent variables', *Annals of Econometrics and Social Measurement,* 5: 493–509.

Olsson, U. (1979) 'Maximum likelihood estimation of the polychoric correlation coefficient', *Psychometrika* 44: 443–60.

Rasch, G. (1980) *Probabilistic Models for Some Intelligence and Attainment Tests*. Chicago: University of Chicago Press.

Rosett, R. N. and Nelson, F. D. (1975) 'Estimation of the two-limit probit regression model', *Econometrica,* 43: 141–6.

Rost, J. (1988) 'Rating scale analysis with latent class models', *Psychometrika,* 53: 327–48.

Schoenberg, R. J. (1989) *LINCS 2.0: User's Guide,* Kent, WA: Aptech Systems.

Schepers, A. and Arminger, G. (1992) *MECOSA: a Program for the Analysis of Mean and Covariance Structures with Non Metric Dependent Variables*. SLI-AG, Frauenfeld.

Schepers, A., Arminger, G. and Küsters, U. (1990) 'The analysis of non-metric endogenous variables: the MECOSA approach', in P. Gruber (ed.), *Econometric Decision Models*. Heidelberg: Springer. pp. 459–72.

Sobel, M. and Arminger, G. (1986) 'Platonic and operational true scores in covariance structure analysis', *Sociological Methods and Research,* 15: 44–58.

Sobel, M. and Arminger, G. (1992) 'Modeling household fertility decisions: a non linear simultaneous probit model', *Journal of the American Statistical Association,* 417: 38–47.

Stewart, M. B. (1983) 'On least squares estimation when the dependent variable is grouped', *Review of Economic Studies,* L: 737–53.

Thurstone, L.L. (1947) *Multiple-Factor Analysis: a Development and Expansion of the Vectors of Mind.* Chicago.

Tobin, J. (1958) 'Estimation of relationships for limited dependent variables', *Econometrica,* 26: 24–36.

11

Researching Population Health: New Directions

Kathryn Dean, Svend Kreiner and David V. McQueen

Introduction

The chapters in this book have taken up contemporary issues in population health research and outlined alternative approaches to health research in populations. There has been no attempt to provide a comprehensive treatment of either theory or methods for population health research. Why then have such a book, and why now? The primary answer to these questions is the widespread perceived need for new types of knowledge to better inform public health policy and practice. Other reasons arise from changes in thinking about theory and methods in science generally – changes that are not yet reflected in the bulk of research and teaching, having to do with health studies conducted on groups or samples or populations.

We are in a period of growing ferment in the field of population health research – ferment about approaches to causation, about the role of theory and about the relationship between theory and methods in scientific research (Wulff et al., 1986; Pearce, 1990; RUHBC, 1989). There is a growing disquiet among population health researchers that something has not been quite right about the way research on health has been conducted. It appears that much health research is driven by a need to satisfy fairly rigid research criteria established much earlier by methodologists concerned with a classical view of science. Many public health researchers argue for adherence to traditional methods of experimental design, randomness, normality and significance, often at the expense of sensitivity and appropriateness to the health research problem being addressed, and without recognition of scientific discoveries pointing to the weaknesses of the traditional approaches. This rigidity is anchored in a scientific paradigm that no longer governs the 'hard' sciences from which it was drawn.

The major problem faced in population health research is how to break away from a rigid orthodoxy which is irrelevant to the special areas of study needed, while at the same time adapting methodologically sound new approaches. A major theme running through the chapters of this book is that research design and methodology should be guided by the purpose of a study rather than by adherence to methodological dogma. The excessive faith placed in experimental research is perhaps the most outstanding example of this problem. Overemphasis on experimental and quasi-experimental designs reflects an outdated approach to pursuing high scientific status. Controlling confounders in order to predict statistical effects of single factors precludes the study of the complex forces actually involved in the preservation or breakdown of human health.

This book presents a new way of thinking about research which is predominantly quantitative and works with large multivariate data sets. There are critical steps to be taken if research in health promotion and public health is to develop further and to take into account the new possibilities inherent in new approaches to study design, data collection and data analysis. Changes are already evident with the widening of the synthesis actually occurring in science and breakthroughs in knowledge about dynamic systems. Stark contrasts between natural and social sciences, between theorists and empiricists, between the analytic and hermeneutic traditions in social sciences are not characteristic of the post-empiricist philosophy of science (Bryant, 1991). The major issue facing population health researchers is not the choice between experimental and partialling approaches to studying causation (see Chapter 1), but a 'crisis of theory – or rather the lack of it' and the need for a better interface between methods and theory (Abell, 1991: 110).

Current thinking about theory to guide research on population health issues is that important dimensions of causation, especially contextualism and dynamism, have been neglected (Kickbusch and Dean, 1992; RUHBC, 1989). In order to introduce these neglected dimensions of the causal forces shaping health, it is necessary to formulate more complex theories. One of the chief arguments of the book is that theory is better specified and improved by appropriate methods. That is, theories can only be revised and reformulated appropriately by multimethod approaches to studying complexity. In quantitative work, this means that interrelationships among essential variables affecting a phenomenon must be understood in order to specify and reformulate theory for subsequent research. Interdisciplinary work is required to develop multimethod traditions of testing and revising theories of health and health behaviour.

Key methodological concerns have to be faced in the development of multimethod approaches to causal research. While not considered directly in this volume, the importance of doing away with the inappropriate and unnecessary conflict between quantitative and qualitative methodological approaches needs greater recognition. It is extremely dysfunctional when these research approaches are viewed as competing or mutually exclusive. This unnecessary divide is finally breaking down. An often destructive defensiveness is dissipating with the growth in sophistication of account-centred methods of analysis (Abell, 1991).

Another key concern revolves around the issue of time in research on health. Dynamic research models demand that the element of time be introduced into data collection as well as the analysis of data. This requires different sources of data and different methods of data collection (Chapters 4 and 5) in addition to theoretical frameworks and new methods of analysis which take into account the dimension of time.

The issue of measurement is often passed over lightly in population health research. Variables of crucial interest – quality of life, perceptions of health, social and physical functioning, social stress, social support, inequality, deprivation, even specific behaviours and morbidity variables – often lack conceptual clarification and specificity. We cannot hope to attain greater understanding of causal processes before addressing the types of measurement issues identified in Chapter 7.

Formulating Theory to Guide Research and Inform Practice

Health research on populations has reached a critical stage. Considerable investment in research on health during the past several decades has yielded an enormous amount of data, but relatively little new knowledge about the role of variables known or believed to influence health. Many of the underlying assertions of public health and health promotion build on statistical associations that are generally not well understood and often become politicized because of their weak scientific base. Strong statistical associations between relative deprivation and poor health, or between specific behavioural habits and health variables, are examples of substantive research areas that need new types of research to elaborate their meanings for public health work.

New ways of collecting and analysing data will hopefully provide firmer and specific understanding of these statistical connections. In order for this to occur, theories which postulate the interrelationships among the types and levels of influences are needed, the type of theory building envisioned by Rosenberg (1968). The original approaches to theoretically guided multivariate modelling in elaboration analysis were lost in the era of routine multivariate statistical modelling based on assumptions of normal distributions and linear relationships. Developments in the natural and physical sciences have pushed the scientific paradigm beyond the simple models of linear science.

The theoretical perspectives arising from the interdisciplinary discoveries in the field of non-linear dynamic systems open the horizons for research on complex systems affecting health. Theoretical frameworks such as the biopsychosocial model and the age-period-cohort (Chapters 2 and 3) illustrate integrative thinking where theory and methods interface in the elaboration of complex systems. Embedding population health research in the study of theoretical domains, as sketched in Chapter 1, would specify the conditions of causation and thus provide more meaningful knowledge for public health policy and practice.

In work on theoretical domains, the relative importance of variables can be studied with different methodological approaches contributing to integrated rather than competitive bodies of knowledge. The problems of counfounding which plague epidemiological analyses and the methods discussed in Chapter 3 would be reduced because the fundamental goal becomes elaboration rather than control. Confounding is never really solved by experimental design or statistical control of other influences. Relationships of interest are simply stripped of the moderating multiple influences that constitute true causation.

Working within the context of theoretical domains allows the researcher to discover the subjects and variables of substantive concern by studying different aspects of the theory with the methods most suited to particular questions which arise in the elaboration of the domain. Account-centred work will often be an important part of this process. In this approach, findings from variable-centred analyses which appear inconsistent can become more readily understood. As pointed out in the discussion of the functions of theory in Chapter 2, fallacious interpretations will be reduced. Substantive clues and insights will become available for specification and modification of the theory.

Advances in Statistical Modelling: Opportunities and Limitations for Population Health Research

Technological advances have created many new opportunities in modern times. However, when used inappropriately technology can make things worse rather than better. In population health research, the development of high-speed computers opened many possibilities for the collection and analysis of population data. At this time it must be asked whether or not the use of computers in population health research represents an advance or a decline in the quality and validity of health research on populations.

An explosion in the collection of data has occurred in most countries. The data are often only presented in descriptive tables, perhaps broken down by age and sex. Statistical packages are misused when data are analysed routinely, without consideration of the appropriateness of the procedures for the research problem, the nature of the data or the mathematical preconditions on which the procedures are based, justifying the criticisms directed towards multivariate statistical modelling.

Superficial analysis of variable-centred data does not suffer only from neglect of theory and problems of model selection. Failure to take on the fundamental scientific work necessary to understand the meaning of variables, the relative influence of intraindividual variability and change, and the stability of variables through time (see Chapter 4, 5 and 6) creates unknown distortions in the results of analyses of variable-centred data and confusion in bodies of research literature. The collection of population data is expensive, and therefore limited economic resources are wasted when data are collected and insufficiently or inappropriately analysed.

The origins of statistical modelling in the elaboration procedures developed for survey research (Lazarsfeld and Rosenberg, 1955; Rosenberg, 1968) emphasized the importance of understanding the nature and direction of relationships, the antecedent and moderating effects of variables influencing a relationship of interest. The major constraint to the elaboration of the meaning of the relationships was the inability to examine all of the relevant variables at one time to study the many relevant interrelationships.

High-speed computers have created new possibilities for moving beyond this fundamental constraint. Yet, in spite of the new possibilities, the nature of the interrelationships is often less well studied than before computers were available. Part of the reason for this may be found in the causal thinking underlying the experimental model, with its focus on removing and looking away from multivariate and moderating influences, but this is not all of the explanation. Educational opportunities for understanding the available procedures and their appropriate use, as pointed out in Chapter 5, simply have not been available to most population health researchers. Some of the most useful procedures for the elaboration of multiple influences have only been available for ten years or so.

Facing Complexity in Population Health Research

It has been known for some time that causal influences are not simple, but the extent of the complexity was not anticipated. Not only is it common rather than exceptional that multiple influences are involved in causing an outcome, but also causal influences often have multiple outcomes (Ory et al., 1992). In order to gain knowledge of this reality, analytic models and techniques must be capable of studying the complex interconnectedness of many types of influences.

The paradigms for what is regarded as proper research in a specific scientific community often include paradigms for what is regarded as proper statistical procedures (Kuhn, 1962). A commonly accepted paradigm will include accepted approaches for building statistical models, for the translation of research problems into statistical terms and for defining the criteria for optimal statistical solutions, for example assumptions concerning parametric simplicity (normal distributions, linear relationships).

Devotion to a specific paradigm in the face of advances in knowledge pointing to inherent limitations in its methods and approaches results in repetition of errors. When new and better solutions are available, adherence to routine use of standard procedures inhibits progress. While this book does not define new and revolutionary paradigms for quantitative health research, it does point to the potential of an approach using theoretical frameworks to guide the collection, analysis and interpretation of results in empirical research. The approach builds on the elaboration of causal processes in contrast to the dominant focus on specific risks.

Elaboration is not limited to variable-centred analysis. Work on a theoretical domain will often involve ethnographic research or work on the interface of macro- and micro-level influences. Data collected and organized as variables for quantitative analyses must spring from theoretically based constructs embedded in knowledge of their complex meanings. In many instances these meanings can only be obtained from in-depth account-centred work.

Understanding intraindividual variability and change (Chapter 4) is a building block in work on a particular substantive domain.

Likewise, exploration of the forces involved in sudden changes in the stability of variables in population data (Chapter 5) can provide insight into the importance of macro-level changes on behavioural and other outcomes at the individual level. It is only the examination of relationships among mutual causes and of the conditions that moderate specific influences which can expand knowledge about the complex causal processes that shape health. An understanding of interactions among numerous level and types of variables is needed for this purpose. The research design and analysis must therefore focus on complexity rather than stripping away the contextual meaning of causation. A multimethod approach, centred in elaborating the real forces shaping health and behaviour, can begin to build bodies of knowledge about dynamic causal processes.

Causal Modelling in Elaboration of a Theoretical Domain

Since the main focus of this book is on quantitative research conducted on population health issues, a closer look at specific issues in the multivariate causal modelling of quantitative data for the purposes of elaborating causal processes can illustrate the integration of theory and methods.

The importance of theory and the consequences for scientific understanding of neglecting theory in empirical work are subjects currently receiving considerable attention in social science (Bryant, 1991). The importance of methods for theory building, as discussed in Chapter 1, is less well recognized. Theory building requires methods that are capable of testing and specifying complex theory, methods which can determine the structure of interactions among numerous types of variables. This means that the statistical methods suited for causal modelling must be able to identify the integral connections between variables in a data set, the interactions and indirect relationships which must be considered along with any correlation between two specific variables of interest.

What we are talking about when we refer to quantitative methods that can contribute to theory building are statistical procedures that can identify the interacting conditions involved in causal complexes in the real world. This of necessity involves multivariate statistical modelling, but, as shown repeatedly in various chapters in this book, multivariate modelling runs into inevitable problems of model choice among huge numbers of possible models. It is easy to take the wrong turn, to create results that are misleading purely because one model was selected over another more correct one:

> the model is subjected to some statistical test. If the test is passed the

> researcher is happy and journal editors are happy and the thing is published. No one likes to mention the millions, billions, or zillions of alternatives that have not been considered, or the dark and troubling fact that among those alternatives there are many which would pass the same statistical test quite as well, or even better, and which would also square with well-established substantive knowledge about the domain. (Glymour et al., 1987).

This takes us to the interface of theory and methods in the elaboration of causal processes described in Chapter 1. The limits of multivariate procedures for causal modelling can only be addressed by using decision aids and rules in the design of the multivariate problems, the model selection in the analytic process and the interpretation of findings (Faust, 1984). These aids involve the careful use of the research literature, and the selection of appropriate statistical models and decision rules for using the procedures in a dynamic interface with theory.

Chapters 6 to 10 of this book discuss statistical models that can be used in this type of interface between theory and methods in the elaboration of a theoretical domain. Two different types of statistical model useful for elaborating complex relationships among variables are discussed in these chapters. One is the class of models for latent structure (Chapter 10), and the other is the class of graphical models (Chapters 8 and 9). The former assumes that unobserved variables explain the variation found in the data, while the class of graphical models makes no such assumption.

Graphical models and latent structure models both build on conditional independence as a basic concept. Both types of model share the property that they create possibilities for the formulation of substantive research theories in the causal modelling process by providing a common framework for the statistical analysis of the numerous variables that should be studied simultaneously in given substantive research areas; this is an important advantage for coping with the dangers of model selection in causal modelling.

In latent structure models, condition independence is often referred to as local independence where it appears as one of several requirements of unidimensionality and validity of indirect measurements. For graphical models the concept of conditional independence is the fundamental building block of the paradigm. All the important properties of graphical models are defined in terms of conditional independence.

Thus these two paradigms for multidimensional modelling include different ideas about how the models should be parameterized. It is customary in latent structure modelling to search for a simple parametric covariance structure. Latent structure models often routinely assume that variables are normally distributed, in which case the proper analysis reduces to a question of analysis of the covariance matrix. The graphical models focus on conditional independence, and are accordingly more concerned with partial correlations and partial covariance structures.

It can be seen that even though both models allow the researcher to study complex multiple influences, the causal thinking behind the two paradigms clearly differs. The differences have to do with opposing views regarding the ability to think in terms of variables which are not or cannot be measured. Some 'realists' reject all concepts of causality that have to do with probabilistic relationships (Wulff et al., 1986). In this form of realism, which is *not* analogous with the idea of studying causal processes as they exist in the real world, both latent variable and graphical models would be rejected. Whatever the position taken on this issue, as pointed out in Chapter 8, if it is not possible to make a direct measurement then latent variable modelling is the only option for proceeding with causal modelling. When it is possible to choose a model, however, certain limitations of latent variable models for elaboration within a theoretical domain must be recognized (for example, see the disadvantages of linear structural equation models outlined in Chapter 9). Models based on simple parametric structures do not allow the elaboration of conditional and moderating influences.

Integrating Theory with the Analysis of Data

The potential of particular statistical models for elaborating complexity does not solve the problem of model choice among the multitude of possible models in multivariate analysis. This is an equally serious problem when using the two types of model discussed in this book. The problem is more serious than simple considerations of model fit and traditional views on confounding.

In Chapter 9, a distinction is made between moderation in the confounding sense and moderation in the interactional sense. The types of misinterpretations and fallacious results that frequently occur with hypothesis testing and automatic search procedures are illustrated. Extending these examples to high-dimensional research problems reveals the magnitude of model choice problems in elaboration decisions.

Knowledge and understanding of the technical analytic issue and options are important, but they cannot solve the model choice problems. Advances in the technical procedures available provide new options for defining recursive structure (Kreiner, 1989) and other types of decision making aids for model choice (Glymour et al., 1987) in the rapidly expanding field of artificial intelligence. These decision making tools are only effective, however, in concert with the dynamic use of theory and existing knowledge in the process of elaboration. This is illustrated in the discussion of the weaknesses of empirical in contrast to substantive statistical models in Chapter 7. Knowledge of prior work in the research domain is an essential aspect of causal modelling, but is still not sufficient, as shown in the example of research on AIDS, for understanding the phenomena studied. Substantive theory is needed to guide model choice and produce findings which can, in turn, contribute to development and modification of the theory in the elaboration of the domain.

Conclusion

Research on population health issues contributes the knowledge base for public health policy and practice. The flowering of classical public health occurred with the discoveries of the social and environmental determinants of health. The rise of positivistic science, along with an almost exclusive focus on specific diseases in the reductionistic biological paradigm that dominated most health research throughout this century, fundamentally affected the development of the field of public health (Kickbusch and Dean, 1992). We now have a great deal of information about the statistical risks associated with specific diseases, but little knowledge about the conditions of risk – the moderating and intervening influences that connect risks to the complex reality that preserves or leads to the deterioration of human health in the real world.

The chapters of this book have taken up issues in research on complexity, and discussed options in research design, data collection and causal modelling for the theory guided elaboration of causal processes. No attempt has been made to provide a comprehensive treatment of the issues faced in causal research, or to cover all of the methodological options for research on complex health questions. Rather, we have attempted to provide an alternative view of causal research, one that recognizes the need for methodological rigour and at the same time the limits of any specific methodological approach. We firmly believe that facing the theoretical and methodological issues, especially the need to integrate theory and the multimethod elaboration of substantive research domains, will provide new knowledge to better inform health policy and practice.

References

Abell, P. (1991) 'Methodological achievements in sociology over the past few decades with special reference to the interplay of quantitative and qualitative methods', in Christopher G.A. Bryant and Henk A. Becker (eds), *What Has Sociology Achieved*? New York: Macmillan.

Bryant, C. (1991) 'Developments in sociological theory', in Christopher G.A. Bryant and Henk A. Becker (eds), *What Has Sociology Achieved*? New York: Macmillan.

Faust, D. (1984) *The Limits of Scientific Reasoning*. Minneapolis: University of Minnesota Press.

Glymour, R., Scheines, R., Spirtes, P. and Kelly K. (1987) *Discovering Causal Structure: Artificial Intelligence, Philosophy of Science, and Statistical Modelling*. New York: Academic Press.

Kickbusch, I., and Dean, K. (1992) 'Research for health: challenge of the nineties', in Shunichi Araki (ed.), *Behavioral Medicine: an Integrated Biobehavioral Approach to Health and Illness*. Amsterdam: Elsevier. pp. 299–307.

Kreiner, S. (1989) *User Guide to Digram: a Program for Discrete Graphical Modelling*. Copenhagen: Statistical Research Unit, University of Copenhagen.

Kuhn, T. (1962) *The Structure of Scientific Revolutions*. Chicago: University of Chicago Press.

Lazarsfeld, P.F. and Rosenberg, M. (1955) *The Language of Social Research*. Glencoe, IL: Free Press.

Ory, M., Abeles, R. and Lipman, P. (1992) 'Introduction', in M. Ory, R. Abeles and P. Lipman (eds), *Aging, Health and Behavior*. Newbury Park, CA: Sage.

Pearce, N. (1990) 'White swans, black ravens, and lame ducks: necessary and sufficient causes in epidemiology', *Epidemiology*, 1: 47–50.

Rosenberg, M. (1968) *The Logic of Survey Analysis*. New York: Basic Books.

RUHBC (1989) *Changing the Public Health*. Research Unit in Health and Behavioural Change, Edinburgh. New York: Wiley.

Wulff, H., Pedersen, S. and Rosenberg, R. (1986) *Philosophy of Medicine*. Oxford: Blackwell Scientific.

Index